McFarlin Library
WITHDRAWN

The Prentice-Hall Dictionary of Nutrition and Health

About the Authors

Kenneth Anderson studied at Stanford University and Northwestern University School of Medicine and served in the U.S. Army Medical Corps. He is a former editor-in-chief of *Today's Health* magazine, published by the American Medical Association, and advisory editor of *Nutrition Today*. He is the author or editor of more than 20 books on health and foods and has contributed articles on medical subjects to *Reader's Digest, Science Digest, Better Homes & Gardens,* and other popular magazines. Anderson also was founder and executive director of the *Coffee Information Institute,* an international clearinghouse of medical and technical information relating to caffeine beverages.

Lois Harmon is president of Publishers Editorial Services, Inc., and a former editor for various reference works, including *Funk & Wagnalls Encyclopedia* and *The World Almanac.* She attended the University of Nebraska and the University of Chicago and obtained much practical experience in nutrition by developing and testing new recipes for several cookbooks.

Kenneth Anderson
Lois Harmon

THE PRENTICE-HALL DICTIONARY OF NUTRITION AND HEALTH

PRENTICE-HALL, Inc., Englewood Cliffs, New Jersey

© 1985 by PRENTICE-HALL, INC.
Englewood Cliffs, N.J.

All rights reserved. No part of this
book may be reproduced in any form or
by any means, without permission in
writing from the publisher.

Printed in the United States of America

Library of Congress Cataloging in Publication Data
Anderson, Kenneth.
   The Prentice-Hall dictionary of nutrition and
health.

   1. Nutrition—Dictionaries.   2. Health—
Dictionaries.   I. Harmon, Lois.   II. Title.
III. Title: Dictionary of nutrition and health.
TX349.A54   1985   613.2'03'21   84–11590

ISBN 0-13-695610-6

ISBN 0-13-695602-5 {PBK}

PRENTICE-HALL INTERNATIONAL, INC., *London*
PRENTICE-HALL OF AUSTRALIA, PTY. LTD., *Sydney*
PRENTICE-HALL CANADA, INC., *Toronto*
PRENTICE-HALL OF INDIA PRIVATE LTD., *New Delhi*
PRENTICE-HALL OF JAPAN, INC., *Tokyo*
PRENTICE-HALL OF SOUTHEAST ASIA PTE. LTD., *Singapore*
WHITEHALL BOOKS, LTD., Wellington, *New Zealand*
EDITORA PRENTICE-HALL DO BRASIL LTDA., *Rio de Janeiro*
PRENTICE-HALL HISPANOAMERICANA, S.A., *Mexico*

Contents

Introduction	ix
Dictionary of Nutrition and Health	1–224
Appendix of Tables	225
Units of Measure	
Abbreviations	227
English-Metric Equivalents	227
Weight, Physical Activity, and Diet	
Approximate Weights of Adult American Men and Women	228
How Increasing Physical Activity Helps Balance Caloric Intake	229
Consumption of Sugar Annually per Person in the United States	229
Caloric Content of Typical American Snack Foods	230
How Adding Fats and Sugar to Foods Changes Their Calorie Count	230
How Freezing and Canning Foods Changes Their Sodium and Potassium Content	230
How Nutrient Values of a Potato Can Change with the Form of Preparation	231
Recommended Daily Allowances (RDAs) and Nutrient Values of Foods	
Recommended Daily Dietary Allowances of Calories and Proteins	232
Recommended Daily Dietary Allowances of Fat-Soluble Vitamins (in International Units)	233
Recommended Daily Dietary Allowances of Water-Soluble Vitamins (in Milligrams)	234
Recommended Daily Dietary Allowances of Minerals (in Milligrams)	235

Contents

Calcium Equivalents of Milk in Various Foods............	236
Protein Equivalents of Various Food Sources............	236
Nutrient Values of Various Cereals (per 3.5-oz. portion).....	237
Cholesterol Content of Various Foods	238
Fat Content and Major Fatty Acid Composition of Various Foods	238
Magnesium Content of Various Foods	239
Potassium Content of Various Foods	240
Sodium Content of Various Foods......................	240

Mineral and Vitamin Sources in Foods

Food Sources of Vitamin A............................	241
Food Sources of Thiamine (Vitamin B-1)................	242
Food Sources of Riboflavin (Vitamin B-2)	245
Food Sources of Vitamin C............................	247
Food Sources of Calcium..............................	249
Food Sources of Iron..................................	251
Food Sources of Niacin (Nicotinic Acid).................	254

Introduction

Eating at home or in a restaurant was a fairly simple matter in the past. Most families, partly as a matter of necessity, grew many of their own fruits and vegetables. They often produced their own chickens as a source of meat and eggs, and almost everyone had friends or relatives with a small farm that could supply fresh milk, beef, lamb, and pork.

Food preparation was also relatively simple and direct, even if a bit more tedious and time consuming. A look at a nineteenth century cookbook, such as *Beeton's Book of Household Management,* shows that one did not require a special vocabulary to understand what might be included in a meal. The ingredients generally included butter, flour, sugar, milk, fruit juices or rinds, spices, and, often for flavoring, a bit of wine or brandy. The dishes certainly were not bland. A vinegar was made with fresh mint leaves, mackerel was served with a gooseberry sauce, a ketchup was flavored with walnuts and port wine, and a sauce for poultry required ½ pt. of melted butter and 3 dozen fresh oysters. There was no reason then to be concerned about BHA and BHT antioxidants, partially hydrogenated soy oil, hydrolyzed plant protein, or monosodium glutamate. Along with FD&C Red No. 40 and aluminum stearate, such items did not exist in the minds and stomachs of the public.

Although meals contained quantities of butter, sugar, flour, and other food items we now consider potentially dangerous to the human body, people of that era who survived the infectious diseases of childhood generally lived as long as the older people of today. The men and women of the past did not participate in jogging or weight lifting for exercise, and their children did not go to tennis camp or basketball camp for fitness lessons. Yet heart disease of the type that claims hundreds of thousands of lives each year in our own era was a relatively rare disorder in the past. But the people of bygone eras simply worked harder at jobs that required greater physical effort. Children walked between home and school rather than being transported in comfort, and they usually worked around the home after school rather than finding relief from boredom in front of a TV screen.

Effects of the American life style on health became obvious during the Korean War. Americans were amazed to discover that Korean soldiers could run up a mountainside that GIs could barely manage in a slow walk. And when doctors examined the bodies of American casualties, they were equally amazed to find the coronary arteries of the hearts of the GIs, many of them still in their teens, streaked with the cholesterol deposits they expected to see only in the hearts of old men. Obviously, something had changed in the health of North Americans. The change appeared to be a heavy price that had to be paid for new ways of living and new ways of eating.

Ironically, in the one or two decades before the Korean War, there had been tremendous progress in the areas of nutrition research and the control of infectious diseases. Most of the vitamins and the antibiotic "wonder drugs" had just been discovered. Scientists were finding ways to use hormones to produce livestock, fruits, and vegetables faster or bigger, or both, than ever before. What should have been the dawn of a golden age of healthful living was clouded by reminders that scientific discoveries and inventions did not guarantee a longer, healthier life unless the information gained could be put to proper use. Indeed, even as nutrition experts were finding ways of fortifying common foods with vitamins, thousands of people were still dying each year of such vitamin-deficiency diseases as pellagra and beriberi. It was nature's way of showing humans that they will always be vulnerable to the ravages of nutritional deficiencies unless they are on their guard.

While some food scientists studied the causes and effects of nutritional deficiencies, others were creating foods that had never existed in nature. In experimenting with new ways to preserve foods so that seemingly fresh fruits, vegetables, and meats might be available to a majority of the people during most of the year rather than just during harvest seasons, the food scientists learned to create illusions of texture, mouth-feel, taste, aroma, color, and other factors from starch, sugar, fat, and a variety of chemical additives. They found, for example, that by adding certain artificial colors to soft drinks or desserts, they could create illusions of sweetness or tartness that were actually in the minds of the consumers and did not require any real changes in the flavoring agents used. A breakfast cereal could be made to appear as a very healthful, crunchy grain product when it consisted of little more than oven-toasted flakes of starch paste. And a raspberry flavor could be created with a mixture of benzyl acetate, methyl butanol, hexyl alcohol, isoamyl caproate, and more than 20 other chemicals.

Thus, the era of processed foods added to the new language of health. After learning the names of vitamins and trace minerals, one had to become acquainted with many strange chemical names in order to know what might replace the simple butter, flour, sugar, and eggs of old-fashioned cooking. The new words were required on food labels by government regulations. And although the government may have been pleased with the new food vocabulary, it is doubtful that the average food consumer had the foggiest notion about the meanings of the BHAs, BHTs, and other terms.

The news media—newspapers, magazines, radio, and television—have also contributed somewhat to the confusion by reporting almost daily on beta-blockers, monoamine oxidase inhibitors, and neurotransmitters, assuming that

Introduction

all readers and listeners would understand without further explanation. A report might announce that people who use monoamine oxidase inhibitors should not drink Chianti wine or eat cheddar cheese because it could result in a tyramine reaction, yet the reporter often lacks the time or space to explain to the public what this really means.

Government agencies also distribute releases and brochures that discuss, for example, the effects of sodium, potassium, calcium, and magnesium electrolytes on the nervous system of women during premenstrual tension. But a young woman who did not study biochemistry in college might fail to appreciate the government's advice. A quasi-governmental agency, the National Academy of Sciences, has warned that certain types of meats might be the cause of stomach cancer because their additives lead to the formation of nitrosamines. Although the report was widely disseminated through the media, it is doubtful that most Americans could explain the chemical relationships between eating a hot dog and developing stomach cancer.

What This Book Will Do for You

The ancient Chinese admonition that health problems should be treated with medicine only when a proper diet fails to produce a cure illustrates a truth forgotten until the 1980s. Before the present decade, it was possible for a physician to become a practitioner of the healing arts without taking a course or reading a single book on the subject of nutrition. Now the great medical schools of the western world have acknowledged an inseparable relationship between a patient's nutrition and his or her physical health. Today, medical schools are beginning to require that candidates for an M.D. degree study nutrition as well.

It would be very difficult to present in one volume an explanation of all the terms currently used in the newly merged nutrition and health sciences. One dictionary that attempts to define all the terms, from the names of herbs to the uses for various dental instruments, contains hundreds of thousands of entries with millions of words requiring several bulky volumes of references and cross-references. *The Prentice-Hall Dictionary of Nutrition and Health* presents a comprehensive selection of the terms that form the basis for a modern language of health in a professional reference guide that is concise, accurate, objective, and authoritative. For the health professional, this dictionary provides in a single volume the essential information about the chemical composition of natural and synthetic foods, food additives and food safety laws, current concepts of clinical nutrition research, the physical effects of dietary deficiencies and excesses, inborn errors of metabolism, and related basic data about human body form and function.

The definitions are written in clear, easy-to-understand language that makes the book equally valuable to the health-conscious nonprofessional who seeks a better understanding of the sources and purposes of the nutrients essential for optimum physical conditioning and increased longevity. Numerous mini-articles

Introduction

describe in detail the roles of vitamins, minerals, fats, proteins, and carbohydrates in human health. This vital information is supplemented with data tables and charts designed to guide the reader to a greater effective use of modern nutrition knowledge. *The Prentice-Hall Dictionary of Nutrition and Health* explains the causes of food allergies, how some foods interact with medicines, and the sources and uses of various artificial flavorings and colorings, in addition to such basic health facts as skin coloring, aerobic exercise, cancer, and heredity. The authors urge you to read the book in good health.

a

abrasion A wound that involves the loss of the outer layer of the skin (epidermis). A deep abrasion into the inner layers of the skin (dermis) may become covered with a blood clot that later develops into a scab.

absorption The process by which simple sugars, fatty acids, amino acids, water, and certain minerals and other substances are extracted from the digestive tract and carried by blood and lymph vessels to the liver for further metabolic activity. Most absorption of nutrients occurs in the small intestine, which is lined with numerous folds and hairlike villi, creating the appearance of carpet pile. These villi, or threadlike protrusions into the intestine, are in constant motion as digested food passes over the folds and wrinkles of the lining.

Villi have thin but highly specialized membrane walls which allow only certain substances to pass through to the lymph vessels inside. A bit of iron may or may not be allowed to pass through the villi wall, depending on such factors as whether the body has received its quota of iron and the way in which the iron is "packaged" with other atoms. Calcium may not be absorbed if it has combined with phytic or oxalic acid to form a compound that will not diffuse through the villi walls. Similarly, protein that has been fried or overcooked may be passed through the intestine without being absorbed because the amino acids have been converted into insoluble substances that cannot be used for building new body tissues.

Absorption is the crucial test stage of an individual diet because the villi make the final "decision" regarding the nutrients that can be used by a person's body and those that are useless or detrimental. Special diets may also have their true test of nutritional value during absorption. If an individual is unable to absorb certain food components, such as the gluten in some cereal products, the condition is called a *malabsorption syndrome,* and is often accompanied by related health problems. One example is vitamin B-12 absorption, which depends on a substance called the *intrinsic factor* which is normally present in the gastric juice. Absorption of both substances in turn depends on the presence of calcium in the intestine. If the body is unable to

1

acceptable daily intakes

absorb vitamin B-12 from the digestive tract, it loses its normal ability to manufacture red blood cells and DNA molecules. See *malabsorption syndrome*.

acceptable daily intakes The daily dose of a chemical used as a food additive that appears to be without serious risk to humans based on the scientific data available at the time.

acerola A small red cherry-like fruit of a plant that grows in Puerto Rico and other tropical areas of the Western Hemisphere. The acerola is reported to contain more vitamin C per weight than any other known fruit or vegetable. Its vitamin C content is approximately 2,000 mg. per 100 g. of fruit,* compared to 50 mg. of vitamin C for an average commercial-grade peeled orange.

acesulfame K An artificial, noncaloric sweetener reported to be about 200 times as sweet as regular sugar. Like aspartame, it was developed for use in dietetic beverages.

acetate A compound formed from acetic acid and a base or alkali substance, or by combining acetic acid with alcohol. One example is potassium acetate, which can be used to correct a potassium deficiency.

acetic acid An organic acid present in varying small amounts in such diverse food products as strawberry juice and molasses. It is the main ingredient in vinegar. Vinegars usually contain between 3 and 5 percent acetic acid. Acetic acid, generally as a vinegar ingredient, is found in catsup, sour pickles, mayonnaise, salad dressings, and certain canned vegetables and cured meats. It is produced naturally by the action of a bacterium known as *Acetobacter aceti* on alcoholic beverages, which accounts for the vinegary aroma and taste of spoiled wine.

acetone One of the acetone bodies formed during the metabolic disorder of acidosis. Acetone is also found in a variety of foods, such as coffee, which derives much of its sweet and pungent aroma from this substance. Because cows often experience acidosis, small amounts of acetone occasionally enter the milk supply, giving it a flavor sometimes referred to as "cowy."

acetone bodies See *ketone bodies*.

acetylcholine A substance composed of acetic acid and choline that occurs naturally in many body tissues but is involved primarily in the transmittal of nerve impulses required for normal body functions. Two types of food

Note: Explanations of abbreviated forms of units of measure used in this book can be found in the "Abbreviations" table on page 227 of the Appendix.

poisoning, botulism and one caused by a shellfish disease, produce their effects by interfering with the secretion of acetylcholine by the nerve cells.

achlorhydria A deficiency of hydrochloric acid in the gastric juice of the stomach. This disorder affects mainly older people who may gradually lose their ability to secrete enough hydrochloric acid to digest food properly.

acid Technically, an acid is a substance that yields hydrogen ions, or positively charged hydrogen particles, in a solvent such as water. The word is derived from the Latin term for "sour," which is a concept that is more easily understood by most people. It is the stimulation of the taste buds by hydrogen ions that gives a food its sour taste. Acids are generally rated according to their proportion of hydrogen ions, as compared with alkaline or base substances. These ratings bear a code, pH, which stands for hydrogen ion concentration. Because of the mathematical formula used, the smaller the pH number the stronger the acid. A pH of 7.0 represents a neutral balance between acids and bases in a substance.

acid-ash diet A diet designed to result in an acid effect in the urine. It usually consists of meats, fish, eggs, and cereals which, when metabolized, yield acidic waste products. An acid-ash diet is sometimes prescribed for persons afflicted with kidney stones. See *alkali-ash diet*.

acid-base balance The balance between the acid and alkaline components of the blood. It must be maintained at a constant ratio to prevent acidosis or alkalosis. The acid-base balance results in a nearly neutral pH value of 7.4. The human body depends on several mechanisms for maintaining a neutral balance, including the rapid excretion of metabolites that threaten to increase the acidity or alkalinity of the blood and body tissues, and by the use of body fluids to dilute substances that might alter the neutral pH value.

acid foods A term generally applied to foods that have a sour taste. Most fruits and vegetables contain one or more weak acids, such as citric, malic, oxalic, or tartaric acid. Lemons, blueberries, and grapefruit are rich in citric acid; cherries, rhubarb, and crab apples contain high levels of malic acid. Acids are often converted to sugar as a fruit matures. They give flavor and color to vegetables and are often dissolved by steam during cooking. Green beans or broccoli cooked in a container without a lid will have a different color than the same vegetables cooked in a covered container to keep the volatile acids from evaporating.

acid-forming foods Foods that contain chemicals which influence the acidity of urine. Foods containing sulfur, phosphorus, and chlorine are acid forming, as are meats, fish, eggs, cereals, and many other protein foods. Milk is an exception to the rule; although it is rich in protein, it is a base-forming food. Many fruits and vegetables, although sour to the taste, are also base forming rather than acid forming because of the chemical transformations they undergo in the body.

acidophilus milk A fermented milk prepared by adding *Lactobacillus acidophilus* bacteria to milk. The milk is prepared in a manner similar to the process used in the manufacture of buttermilk or yogurt, except for the strain of bacteria added. Acidophilus milk is sometimes promoted as a beverage that can have significant health effects by altering the type of bacteria in the digestive tract; however, these claims have been challenged by other nutrition experts.

acidosis A health disorder caused by an accumulation of acids or a depletion of normal alkaline reserves in the blood and other tissues of the body. Acidosis usually occurs as a complication of another health problem, such as diabetes or hyperthyroidism, but mild cases can also develop from fasting or certain fad diets. Symptoms may begin suddenly with vomiting or diarrhea, muscle twitching, abnormal heart rhythm, or feelings of mental confusion. The acidosis patient may also have a fruity breath odor from the acetone that has collected in the body tissues. Also called *ketosis*.

acne A skin disorder in which the oil glands become inflamed when the openings become plugged. The glands are usually located at hair follicles and appear as blackheads or small red lesions, such as pimples. Although acne is frequently blamed on diet factors, there is little scientific evidence to support the claim. More important influences are hormones and improper skin care. Acne in girls is sometimes relieved by female sex hormones. However, they cannot be used in the treatment of male acne without the risk of adverse side effects. When bacterial complications are involved, antibiotics may be prescribed. Control of bacteria is important because they produce an enzyme that converts the trapped skin oil into acids that spread beneath the skin surface and cause severe inflammation.

ACTH An abbreviation for the medical term *adrenocortico-tropic hormone*, a substance produced by the pituitary gland. ACTH can also be manufactured synthetically by stringing together a chain of 39 amino acids. Its natural role is to trigger the release of other hormones by the adrenal glands when the body is subjected to stress. ACTH is also involved in the release of fatty acids from the body's fat deposits when energy is needed quickly, as during an emergency, since fatty acids can be easily converted by the body to glucose molecules to stoke the furnaces of tissue cells.

active tissue mass The aspect of body weight concerned with energy consumption, calculated as the difference between total body mass and the relatively nonactive mass of fat, bone-mineral, and extracellular fluid.

activity   Biological equivalents of various forms of a given nutrient, such as vitamin A activity. It is also used with reference to enzymes. Other synonyms are *potency* and *biological efficiency*.

acupuncture   The Oriental art of inserting needles through the skin in the treatment of physical and mental disorders. Acupuncture is believed by some experts to have started before recorded history, when primitive warriors observed that an arrow wound in one part of the body resulted in health effects in another.

A Chinese manuscript written about 400 B.C. described acupuncture in terms of Taoist religious philosophy, which teaches the need for a balance of forces in nature. The function of acupuncture, according to Taoism, which also introduced the Yin and Yang concepts of universal harmony, is to restore the balance of forces within the body by either stimulating or calming an organ system.

According to acupuncturists, each organ system of the human body is associated with a *meridian*, or energy pathway, that flows beneath the skin. Thus, if the toe and the head are connected by the same meridian, a headache can be treated by inserting an acupuncture needle in a toe. There are at least 12 meridians and 360 acupuncture points. The specific acupuncture point is determined by a diagnosis that involves taking a total of 12 pulse readings, listening to the patient's voice, and examining the skin color.

The needles are usually made of stainless steel and inserted at an angle in a pinched fold of skin to avoid hitting a nerve or blood vessel. Although western doctors are skeptical of acupuncture claims, one scientific explanation for its benefits can be based on the fact that many body tissues rotate, fold, and otherwise change positions during embryonic life. As a result, meridians may be established in the embryo even though they cannot be observed in the adult.

acute   Something that is sharp and sudden, such as a severe pain in the abdomen caused by an obstruction or perforation of the digestive tract. An acute illness is usually one that is severe but of short duration, as distinguished from a chronic illness.

acyl carrier protein   A substance in the body that utilizes molecules of pantothenic acid to synthesize fatty acids.

Adam's apple   See *laryngeal cartilages*.

adaptation   Modification of physiological processes in organisms resulting from changes in environment, food, or nutrient supply.

addiction An ambiguous term often used to describe a condition of psychological and physical dependence on a chemical substance, such as alcohol or morphine. Many drugs that are potentially addictive have important therapeutic value as sedatives, pain killers, or anesthetics, but can have harmful effects if used without proper controls. Most addictive substances are "downers," which depress the central nervous system even though the user may believe they have a stimulating effect. Symptoms of addiction include the need for increasingly larger doses of a drug to obtain the same pleasurable effects, symptoms of illness when the supply of the drug is suddenly interrupted (withdrawal effects), and a craving for the substance that may lead to immoral or illegal behavior in order to obtain a supply.

adenosine triphosphate An energy-rich organic compound required in numerous life processes. It is involved in the active transport, or movement through cell membranes, of various molecules essential for metabolism, is the source of energy needed to convert glucose into carbon dioxide and water, and is used in the synthesis of proteins from amino acids. Abbreviated *ATP*.

adequacy The relationship between the physiological needs of the body and a given intake of a specific nutrient, expressed, for example, as vitamin A adequacy.

adipocytes Special fat cells found in the body. Obese people usually have more adipocytes than those who are thin.

adipose tissue The layers of fat cells distributed throughout the body. The number of fat cells in an individual is generally established in early childhood by infant feeding practices and does not change in later life, although the size of each fat cell may change with the caloric intake of the person. A person who consumes more calories than he burns in daily activity develops large fat cells, which may diminish in size when food intake is curtailed. The pattern of distribution of fat cells may vary with different individuals. The term is derived from the Latin word *adiposus*, meaning "fatty."

adrenal glands Small masses of tissue located on top of each kidney. Each adrenal gland is actually two hormone glands enclosed within the same capsule. One "gland" produces aldosterone and hydrocortisone, which are involved in water and electrolyte balance in the tissues and in making nutrients available to the tissues; it is also a source of male and female sex hormones. The other produces adrenaline, (or epinephrine) and noradrenaline (or norepinephrine), which affect the actions of the heart, blood vessels, and muscles.

Adrenalin The trademark for a synthetic form of the hormone adrenaline (epinephrine) that is used as a medication to relieve symptoms of allergic reactions and also as an emergency heart stimulant. Adrenalin is also the British spelling for the generic term *adrenaline*. See *epinephrine*.

adrenaline A common term for the hormone *epinephrine*. See this entry.

aerobic A term meaning literally "with oxygen." This word is commonly used to describe a type of physical exercise that requires increased oxygen intake and blood circulation, to distinguish it from exercise that is less demanding or which may be performed without accumulating an oxygen debt. A person who has developed a heart and lungs that permit endurance-type exercises, like jogging, without huffing and puffing, is said to have achieved a steady state of aerobic conditioning.

aerophagia Another term for *air-swallowing*. Some people swallow air automatically because of nervousness or other psychic factors; others gulp air with their food or drinks. Aerophagia also occurs with gum chewing. In most cases, the act of air-swallowing results in stomach gas, which is relieved by belching.

aflatoxin A poison produced by several strains of mold that grow on peanuts, cereal grains, green coffee beans, and other agricultural products. Aflatoxin-contaminated feeds can kill poultry and other farm animals and the substance has been shown to cause liver cancer in laboratory animals. Because aflatoxin is carcinogenic, foods known to be contaminated by this mold poison cannot be sold in the United States. Most cases of human aflatoxin poisoning have occurred in warm, humid climates where molds thrive.

afterbirth See *placenta*.

agar A gelatin substitute prepared from several types of seaweed that grow in the Pacific Ocean and adjacent waters. It is an odorless, colorless, transparent gel which is harmless to most people. Agar is used as a stabilizer and thickener in commercial beverages, ice creams, custards, sherbets, jellies, and bakery products. It is a solid at human body temperature and melts at the boiling point of water. Among other uses, it is a component of bulk laxatives.

aging The process of growing older. Aging usually implies gradual changes in the structure of the organism, such as loss of elasticity of lung tissue, replacement of muscle tissue by fat deposits, impaired circulation, or loss of natural teeth. The rate of aging actually varies with different individuals, depending on such factors as heredity, lifestyle, and exposure to environmental risks.

alanine One of the nonessential amino acids that occurs naturally in many proteins. Alanine can also be produced in the muscle tissues from pyruvic acid, a waste product of carbohydrate metabolism.

albumin A sulfur-rich form of protein found in nearly all animal tissues and in many vegetable tissues. Albumins are distinguished from other types of proteins by the fact that they coagulate when heated and can be dissolved in water. Eggs are a common source of albumin, as are peas, wheat, and soybeans. Human blood is a source of albumin that can be processed for use in the treatment of shock victims and in the management of certain cases of malabsorption syndrome.

alcohol A term that usually refers to ethyl alcohol, although there is a large number of substances, from liquids to waxy solids, that can be called alcohol. Glycerin and cholesterol are technically alcohols. Ethyl alcohol, the kind found in whiskey, wine, and beer, is produced through the fermentation of sugar by yeast. When cereals are used to produce alcohol, their starch content must first be converted to sugar by a malting process. The alcoholic content of beverages ranges from 3.5 percent for beer to 55 percent for gin, vodka, whiskey, rum, and brandy.

alcoholism and nutrition Abuse of alcoholic beverages can result in a wide variety of nutrition-related disorders, the most common of which is cirrhosis of the liver. Liver damage is usually a direct effect but the condition may be exacerbated by malnutrition, which is also common among alcoholics who depend on the calories in alcohol as a source of energy. Liver damage in turn can interfere with the body's sugar-starch storage mechanism, resulting in hypoglycemia. Malnutrition and the effect of alcohol on B vitamins in the body often result in deficiencies of thiamine and other B vitamins. Alcoholics also have deficiencies of potassium, magnesium, and zinc.

aldosterone A hormone produced by the cortex of the adrenal gland. It is the principal mineralocorticoid of the body, regulating the levels of sodium, potassium, and water in the blood and other body tissues.

alfalfa A deep-rooted farm crop grown as food for livestock and consumed as seed sprouts by people. Some nutritionists claim alfalfa sprouts provide more protein per serving than an equal amount of beef, plus most of the vitamins and minerals essential for maintaining optimum health. Alfalfa is also reported to be one of the very few plant sources of vitamin B-12. The plant is said to have originated in the Middle East; the Arabs began adding alfalfa to their own diets when they observed that the finest of their horses were those that ate the bushy, green plant.

algal extractives Products prepared from various kinds of algae and seaweed.

algal proteins Protein-rich products prepared from various kinds of algae.

alkalosis

algarroba An alternative term for carob, derived from the Arabic *al-kharrubah*. Algarroba is the word occasionally used to identify the powdered form of carob, which resembles cocoa powder.

algin An alternative term for sodium alginate, a gelatinous substance extracted from a giant brown kelp seaweed that grows in shallow Pacific Ocean waters. It is also manufactured in a powdered form for use as a stabilizer in ice creams, custards, bakery products, and frozen ices. Algin prevents ice-crystal formation in frozen desserts and provides a creamy texture. Pressurized cans of whipping cream often contain algin as an additive.

alimentary canal An alternative term for the digestive tract. It consists of all the organs along the route taken by food passing through the body, from the mouth to the anus

alimentary pastes Macaroni, noodles, spaghetti, and similar products prepared from durum wheat flour with a high gluten content. Also called *pasta*.

alkali Any of a large number of chemical compounds that will react with acids to form salts or with fats to form soaps. Alkalis usually have a bitter taste, as opposed to the sour taste associated with acids. Alkalis are important in the acid-base balance of body chemistry, playing the primary role in neutralizing acids and helping to maintain a blood pH slightly on the alkaline side of the balancing act, which is normal for the human body.

alkali-ash diet A diet planned to result in an alkaline residue in the urine. It consists mainly of fruits, vegetables, nuts, and milk, which yield an alkaline "ash" when metabolized, and a restriction on meat, fish, eggs, cheese, and cereals. Cranberries, plums, prunes, corn, and lentils are also restricted because they are acid-producing fruits and vegetables.

alkalizer A substance that makes something alkaline or that neutralizes an acid. The term may be used to identify a medication that is taken to neutralize excess stomach acid.

alkalosis A disease condition in which there is an accumulation of alkalinity, or base, in the blood and other body tissues, or an abnormal loss of acidity. The condition can result from severe vomiting or use of diuretic medications, among other causes. One common cause is excessive use of antacid stomach remedies. The patient may experience muscle twitching and weakness, irritability, and confusion. Breathing becomes slow and shallow as the lungs attempt to compensate for the condition by increasing the carbonic acid content of the tissues. Alkalosis is the opposite of *acidosis*.

allergen Any substance recognized by a person's body tissues as foreign, or "nonself." Thus, a kidney transplant, blood transfusion, or mosquito bite may produce the same reaction as an invasion by bacteria or viruses or ragweed pollen. The allergen will be attacked by antibodies produced by the person's tissues, causing a release of histamine and other cell chemicals, with effects ranging from local swelling or sneezing to severe shock. People who are extremely sensitive to chemicals in certain foods, particularly children, may react with a rash, gas, diarrhea, asthma, or other effects that may be mistaken for a cold or influenza.

allergy Any individual hypersensitivity to a substance that may be harmless to other people. An allergy makes itself known through an allergic reaction, when a person's tissues release antibodies to attack and destroy the allergen, or chemical in the substance, that is the source of sensitivity. An allergy may appear as symptoms of hives, eczema, asthma, head cold, digestive upset, itching, and, in very severe cases, anaphylactic shock, which can be fatal. An allergic reaction does not occur on the first contact with an allergen because antibodies have not yet been produced; however, antibodies manufactured after the first contact are available to resist any future entry into the body by the same chemical substance.

allicin A volatile sulfur compound that contributes flavor to certain foods. A common source of allicin is garlic. When a garlic bulb is crushed an enzyme produces allicin, which quickly breaks down into another substance. Chemical cousins of allicin give flavor and aroma to onions, horseradish, mustard, and coffee.

allopathy A system of treating disease by producing effects that are different from or the opposite of the symptoms. Most modern physicians practice a type of medicine that is an outgrowth of allopathy. The original allopaths would administer a medication that might produce a fever or nonspecific inflammation to counteract the symptoms of an infection.

allowances A general term for the amounts of food or nutrients recommended for daily consumption by an adult individual. They are usually expressed in practical terms, such as quantities of food or specific nutrients, with a margin of safety above physiologically determined requirements taken into account. See *Recommended Dietary Allowances*; *U.S. RDA*.

aloe extract A bitter juice obtained from any of several varieties of *Aloe* plants that grow in Africa and the West Indies. It is used in very small amounts in flavorings of alcoholic beverages, such as vermouth and bitters. Large amounts of aloe can have serious adverse effects on the digestive system because of its cathartic potential.

alopecia A type of baldness in which there is a loss or thinning of hair caused by illness or other factors rather than an inherited balding pattern. One type of alopecia, called *alopecia cachectica*, is associated with nutritional disorders.

alpha-tocopherol One of several kinds of tocopherol, which is another name for vitamin E. Of the various tocopherols, the alpha version has the greatest activity. Because in early studies of vitamin E, alpha-tocopherol was found to improve the fertility of laboratory rats, it became known as the antisterility vitamin. However, the fertility effect of alpha-tocopherol has not been demonstrated in humans. The word tocopherol is derived from the Greek *tocos*, meaning "childbirth." See *vitamin E*.

alpha-tocopherol acetate The name of a form of vitamin E that occurs in most vitamin supplements. It is derived from alpha-tocopherol, the most active of the various vitamin E sources. Also called *alpha-tocopheryl acetate*.

alum The shortened name of *aluminum potassium sulfate*, a colorless, odorless, crystalline material that may appear as a white powder. It is used to clarify sugar, as a bleaching agent carrier, a hardener of gelatin, and as a firming agent in foods. Alum is contained in baking powder, sweet and dill pickles, bleached and cereal flours, and cheeses.

aluminum A silvery-white metal found in small amounts in human body tissues and in the food supply. However, nutrition scientists have not determined whether it is necessary for normal body functions or otherwise helpful or harmful. Aluminum may enter the life processes simply because it is one of the most abundant elements in the environment, comprising 8 percent of the earth's crust.

aluminum ammonium sulfate A food additive used in baking powders and cereal processing. It is also used to purify drinking water. The odorless, colorless crystals have buffering and neutralizing qualities. The pure chemical, which is also used as an astringent and styptic medication, can cause a burning sensation in the mouth and throat if swallowed in significant amounts.

aluminum calcium silicate A relatively harmless food additive used as an anticaking agent in table salt and powdered vanilla.

aluminum hydroxide A food additive used as a leavening agent in bakery products. Aluminum hydroxide is also an ingredient in certain antacid medications.

aluminum phosphide A fumigating chemical applied to certain processed foods. Because it reacts with moist air to produce a highly toxic gas, phosphine, foods treated with aluminum phosphide must be aerated for 48 hr. before they are offered to consumers and before foods containing more than 1 part per 100-million of phosphine can be sold to the public.

aluminum stearate A plastic-like material used as a component of chewing gum and as a defoaming agent in the processing of sugar beets and yeast.

aluminum sulfate A food additive used in processing fats and oils, pickles, and food starch. Also called *cake alum; patent alum.*

aminoacetic acid See *glycine.*

amino acid An organic chemical compound that occurs naturally in plant and animal tissues and is a building block for protein molecules.

There are more than 20 different kinds of amino acids, most of which can be produced by the human body. However, at least eight of them cannot be produced by the body tissues and must be obtained from foods. They are: isoleucine, leucine, lysine, methionine, phenylalanine, threonine, tryptophan, and valine. A ninth amino acid, arginine, is required for normal infant development and a tenth, histidine, may be needed in the adult diet. Amino acids that cannot be manufactured by the body and must be included in the diet are called *essential amino acids.* Essential, in this case, does not mean the other amino acids are not needed for normal body functions, but rather that it is essential that amino acids not manufactured by the body be included in the foods eaten regularly.

The various amino acids vary in size, structure, and food sources. What they have in common is a pair of chemical components that give the substances their name: an amino portion, consisting of a nitrogen atom and two hydrogen atoms (NH_2), and an organic acid portion consisting of a carbon atom, two oxygen atoms, and a hydrogen atom (COOH). Because of the amino portion, amino acids are the major source of nitrogen for the body and the means by which the body can manufacture other amino acids, by taking the nitrogen atom from essential amino acids in the diet. Carbohydrates and fats do not contain nitrogen.

Very few foods provide all of the essential amino acids. A protein that contains all the essential amino acids is known as a *complete protein.* Probably the best example of a food source of complete protein is the ordinary chicken egg. Most other foods lack one or more of the essential amino acids, or contain inadequate amounts of certain amino acids. For example, soybeans have as much lysine as eggs but lack methionine. Corn, on the other hand, has more methionine than soybeans but is an inadequate source of tryptophan, an amino acid that soybeans contain in high levels. For persons who may be allergic to eggs, or who prefer a vegetarian diet, it is important to know which combinations of meats and/or vegetables to eat in order to be sure of having a diet that provides proper amounts of the essential amino acids.

amino acid chelates Minerals, such as iron, that are absorbed from the digestive tract only after they become bound in a chemical complex, called a *chelate*, with amino acids. Vitamins, particularly vitamin C, may also be involved in the formation of chelates.

amino acid hydrolysate See *protein hydrolysate*.

amino acid reference pattern A theoretical ideal combination of amino acids that are in the proper proportion and total amount to meet all of the body's physiological needs for protein. Although it does not exist in nature, the amino acid reference pattern is used as a standard for determining the minimum nitrogen and amino acid needs of a person.

ammonia A colorless alkaline gas with an acrid flavor and a pungent odor. Ammonia is involved in the manufacture and metabolism of many organic molecules, including the amino acids, because it carries the nitrogen atom. Ammonia combines with carbon dioxide in the formation of urea, which is secreted in the digestive tract and enters the bloodstream. When the body contains large but normal amounts of ammonia compounds, some may be excreted onto the skin in sweat that has a peculiar odor. Ammonia compounds are often used as food additives.

ammonium bicarbonate An alkaline chemical compound used as an additive in certain food processes, mainly bakery products. The gas generated by ammonium bicarbonate when heated improves the volume of eclairs and cream puffs. It is also used in commercial cookie baking because the ammonia released in the decomposition of ammonium bicarbonate when heated adds a flavor and alkalinity touch to the products. Ammonium bicarbonate is seldom used in home cooking because it is very difficult to store and decomposes when warm into carbon dioxide, ammonia, and water, leaving no residue.

ammonium carbonate A chemical cousin of ammonium bicarbonate that is also used in commercial baking processes to produce gas in batters and help control flavors and acidity.

ammonium chloride An ordorless white powder used as a dough conditioner and as a nutrient for yeast cells. Also called *ammonium muriate; sal ammoniac*.

ammonium phosphate See *monobasic ammonium phosphate; dibasic ammonium phosphate*.

amphetamines A group of stimulant drugs that have been used as "pep pills," weight-reducing medications, and by athletes to relieve feelings of fatigue. Amphetamines have also been used therapeutically in the treatment of certain central nervous system disorders, such as epilepsy. They function by releasing stored epinephrine (adrenaline) in the nerves, causing increased activity of various organs and glands. As drugs of abuse amphetamines can be quite dangerous, causing agitation, sleeplessness, tremors, and in some cases, symptoms of schizophrenia or other psychotic behavior.

amygdalin   A potentially toxic substance present in almonds and seeds of certain other plants. An enzyme called *emulsin* can split amygdalin into oil of bitter almond and hydrocyanic acid. Amygdalin is also known as Laetrile, a controversial cancer medication that has been rejected by the U.S. Food and Drug Administration because of its toxicity and the lack of evidence to support its value as a cancer-controlling agent. Also called *vitamin B-17*.

amylase   A type of enzyme that helps the body digest starch by breaking the starch molecules into sugar units. *Pytalin*, secreted by the salivary glands, and *amylopsin*, secreted by the pancreas, are amylases of the human digestive tract. Amylases also occur in other organisms, including plants, where they perform a similar function of converting starches to sugars. Starchy cereals must usually be cooked before amylases in the human digestive tract can convert them to sugars.

amyl flavorings   Any of a number of natural and synthetic flavorings used in beverages, candies, bakery products, gelatin desserts, ice creams, chewing gums, and other items. Examples include *amyl octanoate*, which occurs naturally in apples but is prepared synthetically as an ingredient of an artificial chocolate flavoring; *amyl alcohol*, which occurs naturally in oranges and cocoa but is made synthetically as part of an artificial flavoring for apple, pineapple, banana, and rum flavorings; and *amyl hexonate*, a synthetic additive used in the manufacture of artificial citrus flavorings.

amylopsin   An amylase enzyme secreted by the pancreas that converts starch to maltose, which is a *disaccharide*. See this entry.

amylose   A very large sugar molecule that is a component of starch. An amylose molecule may be composed of several hundred to several thousand glucose molecules strung together in a chain. The amount of amylose in starch varies with the type of food item; for example, about 70 percent of the starch in wrinkled peas is amylose.

anabolism   The building-up of tissues, such as muscle tissue. The term is generally used to describe the body processes in which proteins are built from various amino acids absorbed from the bloodstream by the tissue-building cells.

anaerobic   A term that literally means "without oxygen." This word is sometimes used to describe exercise routines in which muscle contractions are not strenuous enough to produce an oxygen debt. It is also applied to certain types of microorganisms that are able to live without oxygen. See *aerobic*.

androgenic-anabolic steroids   A group of male sex hormones that enhance the body's ability to build muscle tissue by causing the body to retain nitrogen, which is essential for protein production. These hormones have been shown to aid in muscle-building in animal experiments and in the treatment of certain health problems associated with protein deficiencies. They are also used by some athletes for muscle-building, although their use is controversial. Steroid use is particularly controversial for young people and women, since these hormones tend to alter the sexual characteristics of females and can interrupt the bone growth of young men. Little is known about the long-range effects of steroids administered to humans.

anemia   Any blood disorder in which there is a deficiency of red blood cells or a lack of hemoglobin caused by a blood loss through bleeding or destruction of red blood cells, or a failure of the body to produce adequate numbers of normal blood cells. There are dozens of different forms of anemia, including sickle-cell anemia, pernicious anemia, cow's milk anemia, Cooley's anemia, and iron-deficiency anemia. Causes range from heredity to infections, injuries, cancer, exposure to toxins, such as carbon monoxide poisoning, or diet.

anethole   A substance that gives anise, fennel, star anise, basil, and tarragon a sweet, aromatic, licorice flavor. It is used as an additive where appropriate in ice cream, candies, bakery products, chewing gum, and beverages.

aneurin   A term used in Great Britain to identify vitamin B-1, or *thiamine*.

anhydrous   A term used to describe anything that does not contain water in any form.

animal proteins   The proteins contained in fish, meat, milk, and poultry. Animal proteins are often distinguished from vegetable proteins because those from animal sources are more likely to contain all or most of the essential amino acids. It is possible to obtain equivalent amino acids in vegetable proteins, but only by eating combinations of certain plant foods.

anise   The seed of a dried ripe fruit of an annual herb, *Pimpinella anisum*, native to Greece, North Africa, and the Middle East. It is also cultivated in much of Europe and India. However, the main commercial source of the oil of anise used in flavorings is *China star anise*, an Oriental evergreen tree. It yields a sweet aromatic smell used in licorice, anise, sausage, ice cream, candies, bakery products, and beverages.

anisole A pleasantly aromatic synthetic food additive used in certain soft drinks, ice creams, candies, and bakery products for its licorice flavor. Anisole is also used in certain wintergreen flavorings.

ankyloglossia A medical term for tongue-tie. A tongue-tied person may have trouble eating or speaking normally because the tongue is literally tied down by a membrane that prevents the proper extension of the tip of the tongue. The condition is congenital, meaning it was present at birth, and is easily corrected in most cases by surgery to cut the membrane.

annatto A yellow to orange-red vegetable dye obtained from the seeds of the *Bixa orellana* tree which grows in Central America. The yellowish pigment in annatto extract is bixin, a carotenoid substance closely related to the vegetable and fruit sources of vitamin A components. Annatto extract is used to color ice creams, butter, margarine, salad dressings, and vegetable oils. Bixin has replaced some of the artificial food colorings that were discontinued at the request of the U.S. Food and Drug Administration.

anorexia A severe loss of appetite, sometimes resulting in a poor state of nutrition that may be life threatening. Anorexia often has a psychological basis, as in cases of *anorexia nervosa* in young women who express an aversion to food in order to maintain a small, slim body build, or *secondary anorexia*, in which a person with a digestive disorder suppresses the appetite because of a fear of aggravating the condition. Drug addiction, alcoholism, and psychological depression may also be causes of anorexia. See *anorexia nervosa*.

anorexia nervosa A pathological condition that occurs mainly in young women, usually of an age between puberty and adulthood, who have an aversion to food. The condition results in a loss of weight and energy, a reduced basal metabolic rate, and other problems, such as amenorrhea. Psychologists interpret anorexia nervosa as the expression of a fear of taking the step from adolescence to a normal female adult sex role; eating normally would lead inevitably to development of the body of a young adult woman who would be expected to assume an adult female sex role. By starving the body, the patient believes unconsciously she can perpetuate adolescence with a small, slim body build.

Some studies also show the condition is most likely to develop as a reaction to inadequate or destructive relationships in goal-oriented upper-middle-class families in which there is strong emphasis on the virtue of a slim, physically fit body but a lack of normal interpersonal communication.

anosmia A loss of the sense of smell. The condition can result from a head injury that damages the olfactory nerves, which serve the sense of smell; an infection; a swelling inside the nose; or a brain tumor.

anoxia The absence or lack of oxygen, a term that is usually applied to a reduction of oxygen in the body tissues below a level necessary to maintain normal functioning. Anoxia can result from anemia, in which the blood lacks the hemoglobin or red cells needed to carry oxygen to the tissue cells; living or traveling in high-altitude areas where the oxygen pressure of the air is inadequate for the body needs; or circulatory disorders marked by impaired blood flow that would normally carry enough oxygen to the body tissues.

antacid A chemical formulation designed to provide relief from the symptoms of gastric distress by neutralizing the effects of stomach acid. There are two general types of antacids: absorbable, such as sodium bicarbonate or calcium carbonate, and nonabsorbable, of which aluminum hydroxide is an example. Absorbable antacids are generally more potent, but continued use can lead to alkalosis. Aluminum hydroxide used alone may cause constipation and is usually combined with magnesium hydroxide which, when used in excessive amounts, can cause diarrhea.

antagonist A chemical substance that interferes with or blocks the utilization of a nutrient, such as a vitamin and antivitamin. See *anticoagulant; avidin.*

anthocyanins A group of pigmented carbohydrates that give red, blue, and violet colors to flowers and fruits. The red color of strawberries, for example, results from the presence of an anthocyanin. Anthocyanins are unique in that the color of the plant material is determined in part by its acid-base balance. The same anthocyanin may appear red in an acidic environment, blue in a base environment, and violet when the balance is somewhere between acid and base. Cooking and canning fruits and vegetables that contain anthocyanins can change the color by altering the acid-base balance of the food.

antibodies Protein molecules produced by the body's immune system for the purpose of destroying foreign substances, or allergens, that enter the body tissues. Each type of antibody is tailor-made to resist a specific foreign agent, which could be a bacterium, a virus, or a tissue transplant, that has broken through the body's defenses before. Each allergen carries a chemical tag or "ID" that can be recognized by the antibody "scouts" each time it invades the body. Once the invader is identified, the immune system manufactures countless antibodies designed to attack and destroy the particular allergen. See *allergen.*

antibiotic   A substance derived from one living organism that will kill another organism. Antibiotics from molds were used by the Chinese 2,500 years ago, but scientific use of them in controlling infectious diseases did not begin until around World War II. Hundreds of antibiotics are known and nearly 50 are used by doctors today. Most antibiotics work in one of several possible ways: some, such as penicillin, attack the cell membranes of bacteria; others, like the sulfonamides, interfere with cell metabolism of disease agents; still others, like the tetracyclines, disrupt the reproductive processes of bacteria.

anticaking agents   Substances added to food products to prevent lumping, such as magnesium carbonate and tricalcium phosphate in table salt, and calcium silicate in baking powder.

anticoagulant   Any substance that suppresses, delays, or prevents the coagulation of blood. Anticoagulant drugs, such as heparin, are administered to prevent the coagulation of blood clots that could obstruct a blood vessel to a vital organ like the brain or heart. Heparin is a fast-acting anticoagulant; one type that works more slowly is the vitamin K antagonist, a category that includes coumarin and indandione. Vitamin K antagonists suppress the manufacture in the liver of four blood-clotting factors that require *vitamin K*. See this entry.

antidiuretic hormone   A hormone secreted by the pituitary gland that signals the kidney to reabsorb water into the bloodstream instead of excreting it in urine.

antihemorrhagic factor   An alternative term for vitamin K, a substance in the diet that controls a series of blood-clotting factors needed by the body to prevent hemorrhage. See *vitamin K*.

antimicrobials   Substances used in food processing that prevent or inhibit the development of microbes.

antioxidants   Substances that prevent or retard the tendency of foods, particularly foods containing fats or oils, from absorbing oxygen from the air. The absorbed oxygen causes the foods to become rancid. Substances used as antioxidants include natural agents, such as ascorbic acid (vitamin C) and tocopherol (vitamin E) and synthetic chemicals, such as BHA and BHT, which may be combined with other substances, including citric acid, depending on the kind of food to be protected against rancidity.

antiperistalsis   The opposite or reverse pathway of peristalsis. The term is sometimes used to describe the activity of the digestive tract that accompanies vomiting or feelings of nausea. The action is caused by waves of muscle contractions that normally move digesting food forward from the esophagus, shifting into reverse gear, which pushes the food back toward the mouth.

antipernicious anemia factor   A term used by nutrition scientists in the early days of vitamin B-12 research to identify the substance now known to be the vitamin itself. It was known that pernicious anemia patients who ate liver daily got relief from symptoms of the disease, but researchers were unable to isolate the active substance in liver that controlled it. Thus, the mysterious substance was called the antipernicious anemia factor, abbreviated *APA*.

antirachitic vitamin   A vitamin that provides protection against rickets. *Vitamin D* is the antirachitic vitamin.

antiscorbutic   A term used to identify an agent that suppresses the symptoms of the vitamin C deficiency disease, scurvy. For most practical purposes, *vitamin C*, or ascorbic acid, is the antiscorbutic agent.

antitoxin   An antibody that reacts to the toxin, or poison, produced by a plant, animal, or microorganism. A plant poison, such as the ricin of a castor bean, is a *phytotoxin*; spider or bee venom is a *zootoxin*; and a microorganism like bacteria may produce an *endotoxin* (inside the cell) or *exotoxin* (outside the cell membrane). Antitoxins are usually obtained from the blood of humans or animals who have developed immunity to the toxin from previous exposure and therefore can produce the specific antibodies to neutralize it.

antivitamin   See *vitamin antagonist*.

apastia   A psychiatric disorder in which a person avoids eating food.

aphagia   A medical term for an inability to eat.

aphrodisiacs   Any agents that stimulate sexual arousal or are associated with sexual excitement. Various foods, aromas, and drugs have been identified as having aphrodisiac effects, but the effectiveness of most has been challenged and many such substances produce unpleasant aftereffects. Ginseng is regarded as an aphrodisiac in the Orient where huge sums are paid for ginseng roots that bear a remarkably close resemblance to humans. Amyl nitrite, a depressant, is used as an aphrodisiac, as are potent stimulants, such as amphetamines and cocaine, which presumably are used because they increase blood pressure and tension of the involuntary muscles.

aphthous ulcer   A medical term for a canker sore, a lesion of the tongue that may be caused by a food allergy, an emotional upset, or a viral infection. The sores may appear singly or in groups of as many as 10 to 15. Recurrent attacks are common and women are affected more often than men.

apoenzyme   A large protein molecule that is one part of an enzyme. It is joined by a second unit, the coenzyme, to form a functioning enzyme. However, each part may occur as a separate entity in body tissues.

appendicitis   An inflammation of the appendix, a tubelike extension of the large intestine. Appendicitis is a serious disease because of the probability that, without immediate treatment, the appendix will rupture, leading to peritonitis from the spread of fecal material throughout the abdominal area. Symptoms of appendicitis include nausea with abdominal pain (usually centered in the lower right area of the abdomen), fever that may be high in children but mild in adults, and possible constipation or diarrhea and vomiting.

appendix   A slender, wormlike structure attached to the large intestine near the point in the lower right portion of the abdomen where the small intestine empties into the larger bowel. The appendix has no function in humans but it can become inflamed by fecal material, worms, or other irritants in the digestive tract, causing the disorder known as *appendicitis*. See this entry.

appestat   A term sometimes used to identify the appetite and satiety centers of the brain. See *appetite center, satiety center*.

appetite   An immediate desire, motivation, or impulse to satisfy a physiological need of the body, a term generally applied to an insistent desire to eat. Appetite is also used to identify the impulse to satisfy thirst, the sexual drive, and a need for air. Although appetite is based on bodily needs, it is influenced by external stimuli, such as the aroma of food, the sight of an attractive meal, the sound of a sizzling steak, and so on. Some psychologists define appetite as hunger for a specific item, such as hunger for a cheeseburger.

appetite center   An area of the hypothalamus, located near the base of the brain, containing specialized nerve cells that can detect changes in the level of nutrients flowing in the bloodstream. These nerve cells are believed to cause internal stimulation of a desire to eat when the amount of glucose or other nutrients in the blood falls below a minimum concentration. See *lateral hypothalamus; satiety center*.

arabinogalactan   A complex sugar compound extracted from wood and used as a nonnutritive sweetener, emulsifier, binder, and stabilizer in certain salad dressings and puddings.

arachidonic acid A highly unsaturated fatty acid essential in the diets of some humans, particularly infants, in order to prevent an eczema-like skin inflammation. It is assumed that most adults have accumulated enough arachidonic acid in their tissues to prevent this skin disorder. Also, the body's chemical processing system can usually manufacture arachidonic acid from linoleic acid, which is more often present in the diet. However, the body cannot manufacture linoleic acid, which is an essential fatty acid. Sources of arachidonic acid include animal fats and most vegetable oils.

arginine An amino acid that is generally nonessential. It is one of two amino acids that are basic, the other being lysine, as distinguished from acidic amino acids, such as glutamic acid, and neutral amino acids, which include tryptophan and phenylalanine. Although nonessential as an amino acid, arginine is necessary for normal health because it detoxifies the ammonia produced by the metabolism of proteins.

ariboflavinosis A disease caused by a deficiency of riboflavin, or vitamin B-2. Symptoms include inflammation and fissures that develop at the angles of the mouth, with encrustation and loss of tissue cells. The corneas of the eyes may become reddened by a proliferation of capillaries and the patient may experience eye fatigue and sensitivity to light. A skin inflammation may develop about the nose and other body areas, such as the genitalia. However, the symptoms are not uniform and few patients of ariboflavinosis have the same physical effects. See *riboflavin*.

arrowroot A tropical American tuberous plant with roots that are a source of a nutritive starch. Arrowroot is about 23 percent starch, with about the same proportion of amylose as white and sweet potatoes. It is favored for use in some foods because it forms a translucent, jelly-like paste when boiled, contributing body without cloudiness to the food item.

arsenic A highly toxic substance that is generally present in the environment because of many years of use of the poison in the manufacture of weed killers, insecticides, paints, wallpaper, ceramics, glass, and medicines. Federal law now limits the amount of arsenic residues in the food supply to 65/100 of 1 mg. per pound of food, which is about 0.005 percent of a lethal dose.

arteries Blood vessels that carry blood away from the heart, regardless of other factors, like whether the vessels carry freshly oxygenated red blood or deoxygenated dark blood. A typical artery has four tissue layers, an endothelial lining covered by an elastic membrane, with both enclosed by two layers of muscle. The outer muscle layer has fibers that run the length of the artery and the inner layer has circular muscle fibers. The muscle and membrane layers give the artery a certain amount of flexibility. The largest arteries in the body may also carry their own supply of nerve fibers and capillaries to support functions of the muscle layers.

arteriosclerosis A general term used to identify several kinds of artery diseases marked by a thickening and hardening of the artery walls. Arteriosclerosis may be caused by accumulations of fibrous tissue, fatty deposits, or mineral deposits, such as those of calcium salts, or a combination of such factors. When the condition is caused mainly by fatty deposits, the disorder is called *atherosclerosis*.

arthritis A general term for about 100 different disorders that involve the inflammation of one or more body joints. The most common types are *rheumatoid arthritis*, which is marked by inflammatory changes in the body's connective tissues and is believed to be caused by a breakdown in the body's immune system; and *osteoarthritis*, or degenerative joint disease, which is caused by wear-and-tear on the weight-bearing joints, such as the hips and knees, and affects almost anyone who lives through middle age. Other kinds of arthritis include gout, amyloidosis, systemic lupus erythematosus, congenital hip dysplasia, and tendonitis.

ascites A disease condition caused by an abnormal accumulation of fluid in the peritoneal cavity of the abdomen, causing distention of the abdomen. Ascites can be a sign of a disease of the liver, such as cirrhosis, or of the heart or kidneys. Treatment usually requires a low-sodium diet that prevents fluid retention and helps rebuild body tissues.

ascorbic acid An alternative term for vitamin C. The word ascorbic is derived from the Scandinavian term *scurf*, or scurvy, meaning "a disease characterized by scars or scabs." Scurvy became Latinized to *scorbutic*, from which ascorbic, meaning literally "antiscurvy," evolved. Scurvy, caused by a deficiency of vitamin C, was an ancient plague of seasons when fresh fruits and vegetables were not available. Medical reports of scurvy appear in stories of the Crusades and early sea voyages. See *vitamin C*.

ascorbyl palmatate A food additive derived from ascorbic acid and used in the processing of meats, candies, and fruits.

ash In nutrition, the mineral content of food. The amount of ash is determined by burning a measured sample of food and weighing the portion that remains, assuming that moisture, fats, carbohydrates, and protein portions were consumed or driven off by the process, leaving only a mineral residue.

aspartame An artificial sweetener developed in the 1960s from an organic compound that combines two amino acids. Because aspartame is 160 times as sweet as an equal amount of sugar, it has been introduced as a low-calorie sugar substitute.

aspartic acid A nonessential amino acid that is acidic and plays an important role in the regulation of carbon dioxide in the tissues. Dietary sources of aspartic acid include a wide variety of plants, particularly those produced for their sugar content. It is also synthesized in the body with the aid of biotin.

aspergillus A genus of fungi that includes species both harmful and useful to people. *Aspergillus auricularis* is used commercially as a substitute for malt in the conversion of starch to sugar; *Aspergillus flavus* and *Aspergillus fumigatus* are sources of antibiotics; *Aspergillus niger* is used in the synthesis of citric acid. However, *A. flavus* is also the source of a poison, aflatoxin, that kills farm animals and is a known cause of cancer, and *A. auricularis* can be a cause of ear infections.

aspirin A pharmaceutical name for a compound also known as acetylsalicylic acid that was introduced in the late nineteenth century as a pain reliever and fever reducer. Aspirin is the most widely used therapeutic agent today; in the United States alone, consumption amounts to an average of 150 tablets per person each year. Salicylic acid, a major ingredient of aspirin, has been known for about 2,500 years as an ingredient extracted from the bark of willow trees for use as a remedy. The other major ingredient, acetic acid, becomes noticeable as a vinegary odor when aspirin has been exposed to the air for too long; this odor is a sign that the aspirin's potency is deteriorating.

assay The analysis of the quantity of a nutrient present in a food, for example, vitamin A assay, relative to a standard of reference.

assimilation In physiology, the incorporation of digested food materials into the tissues of the organism. The process usually involves the conversion of digested food into a turbid yellowish fluid, called *chyle*, that can be absorbed through the hairlike projections lining the intestine and transported to the liver and other organs for further processing and utilization.

asthma A respiratory disease in which the person has difficulty exhaling normally. The disorder is marked by spasms of coughing caused by contractions of the bronchial muscles and the presence of fluid obstructing the nasal passages. Because of the bronchial spasms, air enters the lungs faster than it can be expelled, causing the lungs to become distended. Asthma attacks are often related to an allergic reaction to house dust or other inhaled allergens, a condition sometimes called *extrinsic asthma*. Asthma attacks not related to allergens are a sign of *intrinsic asthma*. Attacks may also be associated with the use of beta-blocker drugs taken to treat a different health problem.

atherogenic diet A diet that is capable of accelerating the formation of atheroma, the deposits in arteries that produce arteriosclerosis.

atherosclerosis A form of arteriosclerosis, or hardening of the arteries, in which the main culprit is an accumulation of fatty deposits on the linings of the arteries. As the *lumen*, or bore, of the arteries narrows from the deposits, the walls of the arteries also lose their flexibility so that normal blood flow eventually becomes restricted or obstructed. In addition to hereditary factors that may increase susceptibility, atherosclerosis is associated with aging and may affect several body areas at the same time, setting the stage for stroke, heart attacks, and intermittent claudication by affecting arteries in the brain, heart, and legs.

athiaminosis A deficiency of thiamine, or vitamin B-1. Thiamine deficiency is generally associated with beriberi, a malnutrition disorder of Orientals who eat polished rice with a diet composed predominantly of carbohydrates. In the Western world, thiamine deficiency may be associated with alcoholism, pregnancy or nursing, hyperthyroidism, or fevers that interfere with normal digestive processes. Symptoms include lack of motivation, loss of appetite, mental depression, irritability, inability to concentrate, and memory deficiencies. Untreated, the condition progresses to neuritis and muscular atrophy, difficulty breathing, enlarged heart, and irregular heart beats.

ATP See *adenosine triphosphate*.

atrophy The progressive deterioration or wasting away of body tissues or organs. Atrophy may be caused by the death or reabsorption of cells, or both, or by malnutrition, loss of ability of the cells to proliferate, or interruption of a normal flow of oxygen and nutrients to the cells by the bloodstream. Atrophy may be associated with fatty infiltration of the tissues, erosion of bone-minerals, and hormonal changes, such as those accompanying menopause. Atrophy of the nervous system is a characteristic of certain inherited disorders.

avidin A protein that occurs in low concentrations in raw egg white. Because it binds biotin and makes it unavailable to the individual, it is classified as an *antivitamin*, or vitamin antagonist. People who eat raw egg whites in quantity run the risk of developing biotin deficiency, marked by muscle pains, loss of appetite, insomnia, mild anemia, and a grayish pallor with a scaly skin inflammation.

avitaminosis A vitamin deficiency disease. The term is usually used with the identity of the vitamin involved, such as avitaminosis A. The cause may be a lack of the vitamin in the diet, an inability of the body to absorb the vitamin from the intestine, or a failure of the body to utilize the vitamin because of another abnormality of the individual.

b

baby foods Foods that are manufactured for use by infants. In the United States, where commercially processed baby foods are commonly used, they are regarded by the U.S. Food and Drug Administration as food for special dietary uses and are regulated to a certain extent by rules requiring the listing of ingredients on the label. *Infant foods*, an alternative term, are prepared in a fine puree; baby foods are strained, and *junior foods* may be prepared in a solid but soft form, or in small soft pieces. Because of the baby's delicate digestive system, strained or pureed vegetables must be smooth, prepared with little or no seasoning, and with as much nutritive value retained as possible. At one time, baby foods were seasoned with monosodium glutamate (MSG) and table salt in order to enhance the appeal to the mother, who tended to judge the infant's tastes by her own. However, MSG and excessive levels of salt have been discontinued in recent years.

bacillus vaginalis A strain of bacteria that occurs in the vaginal tract and is a cousin of the *Lactobacillus acidophilus* used in the manufacture of acidophilus milk. The Lactobacillus family encompasses numerous bacterial strains associated with human nutrition and physiology, including several types found in the intestine, used in making yogurt, and which cause tooth decay.

bacteria The plural of bacterium, any of a vast group of microscopic plants found throughout the environment, in soil, water, organic matter, or the bodies of plants and animals, including humans. Some types of bacteria cause disease but most are not harmful to humans and more than a few strains are beneficial.
   All bacteria are one-celled organisms and are classified into three main categories according to their shape. The rod-shaped bacteria are identified as *bacilli*, the spiral-shaped are *spirochetes*, and the roundish type are called *cocci*. The cocci are further classified according to the manner in which they form groups. Pairs of cocci are called *diplococci*, those that form chains are *streptococci*, and cocci that live in bunches are known as *staphylococci*. Staphylococci are usually found on the skin surface of humans, but may produce an infection by entering a break or cut in the skin. Streptococci tend to

enter the bloodstream and spread a serious infection throughout the body. Diplococci usually enter the body through the mouth and nose and may infect the lungs or central nervous system. Gonorrhea is caused by a cocci species and syphilis is caused by a spirochete, but both usually invade the body through the genitalia. Bacilli are less specialized and cause a wide variety of diseases, including leprosy, tuberculosis, and bubonic plague.

Among helpful bacteria are strains of streptococcus used in butter processing to enhance the flavor. Bacterial proteins help synthesize proteins from carbohydrates or other units of carbon and hydrogen. Several strains of bacteria are involved in the synthesis or absorption of vitamins and other nutrients.

bacterial proteins Proteins produced by bacterial action on other substances, such as carbohydrates or other molecules containing amino acid elements.

bacterial toxins Poisonous substances produced by bacteria and the cause of symptoms of a number of serious kinds of infectious diseases and food poisonings. One form of bacterial toxins, exotoxins, are the most poisonous substances known. They are formed and excreted by bacteria into their environment and remain potent even after the bacteria have been removed. Examples include the toxins of diphtheria, tetanus, and botulism. Endotoxins are bacterial toxins found within the cell membranes of bacteria and include those produced by tularemia, bubonic plague, and brucellosis, a group of animal diseases transmitted to humans from livestock.

baker's yeast A yeast that is usually a mixture of special strains of yeasts, sometimes containing strains of *Lactobacillus* bacteria, with the ability to ferment flour-dough carbohydrates. The fermentation process yields carbon dioxide gas which becomes trapped by gluten, the protein portion of the wheat flour, causing the dough to rise. See *brewer's yeast; yeast*.

baking powder A leavening agent used to increase the rate of rising of dough in baking processes. A baking powder usually contains a mixture of chemicals, such as sodium bicarbonate and sodium aluminum phosphate or tartaric acid, which react to produce carbon dioxide gas. The gas accounts for the dough-rising effect.

baking soda See *bicarbonate of soda*.

balance The metabolic relationship between the intake and excretion of a specific nutrient. The word may be combined with the name of the nutrient, such as *calcium balance* or *nitrogen balance*. It may also be used to indicate retention in the body of the nutrient, which would be *positive balance*, or a rate of excretion exceeding intake, which would be *negative balance*.

balanced diet An ideal diet with the appropriate proteins, fats, and carbohydrates included in the proportions required by the body. The term has been both modified and abandoned in recent years by various nutrition experts as new knowledge about micronutrients has been acquired and the theoretical concept of a perfect diet has become more difficult to achieve on a regular daily basis from natural foods alone. See *basic food groups*.

barbiturates A group of potent sedative and hypnotic drugs consumed in the United States alone at a rate of 1 billion doses per year. About 20 different types of barbiturate drugs are used by physicians for various patient needs; each has a somewhat different sedating or hypnotic effect. These drugs are highly addictive and account for more than 1,500 fatal overdoses each year. Barbiturates are named for Saint Barbara because they were discovered on the day when Christians honor this saint.

barium A metallic element that occurs in chemical compounds used in pesticides, paint pigments, fireworks, and other products.

Barium is also used in a sulfate compound administered for x-ray examination of the digestive tract. The element blocks the passage of x-rays through organs coated with it and thus forms a detailed outline of enlarged organs, tumors, peptic ulcers, or other defects. When administered orally, the barium sulfate is mixed with water and a flavoring and called a *barium meal*. A similar solution of barium sulfate is administered through the rectum as a *barium enema* for detailed examination by x-ray of the colon. The sulfate form of barium is insoluble and relatively safe if it has not been contaminated during manufacture by soluble salts of barium, which can be quite poisonous.

The average adult body contains around 3 parts per 10-million of barium acquired from the environment; 1 g. of barium in the body would prove fatal. In some areas, public drinking water supplies have been contaminated by barium, making the water dangerous for use in dialysis equipment or in the preparation of baby formulas. An excessive intake of soluble barium can result in abdominal pain, difficult breathing, paralysis, and cyanosis, a condition in which the individual's skin develops a bluish tint because of lack of oxygen in the blood.

basal metabolic rate A measure of a person's oxygen consumption when he is awake but at complete body rest. The figure may be expressed in calories, assuming that each liter of oxygen consumed is equivalent to slightly less than 5 calories. The person is required to avoid food for at least 12 hr. before the test, as well as muscular exertion for the previous hour. Other factors, such as noise and temperature extremes, that might affect a person's physiology during the test are also avoided. Age, sex, body weight and height, race, occupation, and other factors may be included in a detailed study of basal metabolic rate. Abbreviated *BMR*.

basal metabolic requirement The number of calories an individual requires to maintain his body's automatic body functions for one day. It does not include the calories needed to do anything that requires physical activity, but only quite literally the calories needed to sustain life while doing nothing more than lying awake in bed. Depending on height, weight, sex, and other factors, a person's basal metabolic requirement averages about 1,440 calories per day. Any activity, such as work, sports, or merely playing cards, requires additional calories.

basal metabolism The metabolic activity required to maintain the automatic functions of the body, such as heart contractions, breathing, blood circulation, digestion, and burning of nutrient fuel in order to produce and maintain normal body temperature. Basal metabolism does not include any body activity that involves voluntary muscle contractions or related functions. Also called *resting metabolism*. See *basal metabolic rate*.

base Any substance that is alkaline in nature, or that combines with an acid to produce a salt. See *acid-base balance*.

base-forming foods Foods that tend to neutralize the acidity of the urine because of the alkalinity of their metabolic by-products. Most fruits and vegetables are base forming because they are rich in potassium and sodium, elements that form alkaline compounds in the body. Milk is a base-forming protein because of its high calcium content. See *acid-base balance; acid-forming foods*.

basic food groups A system of organizing food sources into categories of either four or seven basic units to help in planning nutritionally adequate diets. The original seven food groups included: (1) yellow and green leafy vegetables; (2) citrus fruits, tomatoes, and cabbage; (3) potatoes and other vegetables and fruits; (4) dairy products; (5) meats; (6) breads and cereals, and (7) butter or margarine. The U.S. Department of Agriculture later revised the system to include: (1) dairy group, (2) meat group, (3) fruit and vegetable group, and (4) bread and cereal group. A number of daily servings from each group assures representation of the proteins, carbohydrates, fats, vitamins, and minerals needed for a nutritionally sound diet.

B-complex vitamins A term sometimes employed to identify all water-soluble vitamins that contain nitrogen. The group includes thiamine, riboflavin, niacin, folic acid, and vitamins B-6 and B-12. Ascorbic acid, or vitamin C, is a water-soluble vitamin but it does not contain nitrogen and therefore is not a part of the B-complex of vitamins. The name B-complex was acquired during the early history of vitamin research when it was believed that there were two kinds of "food hormone" factors, a "fat-soluble A," which eventually became vitamin A, and a "water-soluble B" factor. When later research disclosed that the substance known as "water-soluble B" was actually a complex of several different water-soluble nutrients, scientists began identifying the various components with numbers, such as B-1, B-2, and so on. Now it is known that except for being water soluble, containing nitrogen, and often occurring in the same food sources, the members of the B-complex group have little in common. Also abbreviated B_1, B_2, and so on.

benzaldehyde An organic compound with a strong flavor of bitter almond. It occurs naturally in bitter almond and is also manufactured synthetically as a flavoring additive for a variety of foods.

benzoate of soda See *sodium benzoate*.

benzoic acid An organic acid present in cranberries, plums, and prunes. Benzoic acid is converted by the liver to hippuric acid, which is excreted in the urine. It also increases the acidity of the urine as an exception to the general rule that fruit and vegetable acids are not acid-forming foods. Benzoic acid may also be used as a preservative.

benzoyl peroxide A bleaching agent used to whiten flour and certain dairy products, particularly cheeses. As the chemical bleaches, it changes into benzoic acid, a common food preservative that is relatively harmless in small amounts. See *bleaching and maturing agents*.

beriberi A disease caused by a deficiency of vitamin B-1, or thiamine, and marked by polyneuritis, fluid retention, and enlarged heart with abnormal heart rhythms.

Beriberi is an Oriental word meaning "I cannot do anything." The disease was described in Chinese medical literature written thousands of years ago. It was once epidemic in Japan, China, India, and Southeast Asia, and was actually introduced to the Philippines by well-meaning Americans who believed that white polished rice was superior to unpolished rice which contained thiamine in the hulls.

The Japanese began the first serious search for the cause of beriberi around 1880, when Europeans believed the disease was caused by a bacteria. The Japanese Navy provided its sailors with polished rice and frequently had 40 percent of its personnel hospitalized with beriberi. British sailors using the same ports ate oatmeal, milk, vegetables, fish, and meat but had no loss of crew members from beriberi. One Japanese doctor required the crew of one ship to eat a British Navy diet and found it prevented beriberi. However, an additional half-century passed before vitamin B-1 finally was isolated.

Beriberi is sometimes separated into two main types. One, called *dry beriberi*, is marked by flaccid paralysis, muscular atrophy, and heart disorders.

The other, characterized by heart failure and fluid retention, but without paralysis, is called *wet beriberi*. Breastfed babies of mothers with beriberi may develop a form of the disease called *infantile beriberi*. Beriberi occurs in North America in alcoholics and persons who fail to include food items rich in thiamine in their meals.

beryllium A metallic element of industrial importance, particularly in the manufacture of aerospace equipment, but which is highly poisonous to humans. Symptoms include respiratory distress, with scarring of lung tissue and heart damage. The condition caused by exposure to beryllium is called *berylliosis*. Beryllium interferes with human metabolic functions that involve the mineral magnesium. It has been used to produce a phosphorescent coating in cathode ray tubes and fluorescent lamp bulbs, although this practice has been discontinued in recent years by most manufacturers because of the danger of exposure to broken tubes and lamps.

beta-blocker A substance that interferes with normal neurotransmitter activity in certain nerve cells called *beta-receptors*. Epinephrine is a beta-receptor neurotransmitter, acting directly on beta-receptors of the heart muscle to increase the heart rate and later its rhythm. An example of a substance that blocks the epinephrine action at the beta-receptor is propranolol, a commonly used heart medication. By interfering with the stimulating action of epinephrine on the heart, a beta-blocker drug can slow the heart rate and reduce the workload on the heart, thereby reducing the risk of angina pectoris, cardiac arrythmias, and other heart disorders. Various beta-blocking agents also are prescribed for the treatment of hypertension, migraine, and glaucoma. Also called *beta-adrenergic blocking agent*.

betaine An organic compound that is present in many plant food sources and can also be synthesized from choline. It is involved in functions of one of the essential amino acids, methionine, and may be used in the treatment of muscular weakness. A combination of betaine and hydrochloric acid is administered to persons suffering from a deficiency of hydrochloric acid in the stomach to increase the acidity of the gastric juices.

BHA An abbreviation for an antioxidant additive chemical with the full name of butylated hydroxyanisole. BHA is used in nearly every food product that contains fats or oils, from lard to processed nuts, to prevent the fatty portion from absorbing oxygen from the air and becoming rancid. See *antioxidants*.

BHT An abbreviation for butylated hydroxytoluene, a synthetic antioxidant used in most processed foods containing fats or oils to extend the shelf life of the product by retarding rancidity. BHT is frequently used as an additive in combination with BHA. See *antioxidants*.

bicarbonate The name applied to the salts formed by the reaction of carbonic acid and a mineral source, such as sodium or potassium. Bicarbonates function in the body as chemical buffers that help maintain the acid-base balance. The carbonic acid from which bicarbonates are formed is merely carbon dioxide dissolved in water, a natural form of seltzer or club soda.

bicarbonate of soda An alternative term for sodium bicarbonate, a salt formed by the reaction of a sodium compound and carbonic acid. See *bicarbonate*.

biceps The main muscle that flexes the arm. The name literally means *two heads* because the biceps has two points of origin in the shoulder area. But the two parts are actually joined in a long tendon that crosses the elbow joint and attaches to the radius, one of the two bones of the forearm. In addition to raising the forearm, the biceps is the muscle that turns the palm upward. When the forearm is flexed, the biceps shortens and expands, producing the bulge of muscle seen on the upper arm. See *triceps*.

bicycle ergometer A stationary bicycle attached to instruments that measure a person's maximum work rate or maximum work output. A bicycle ergometer can be used to determine the effects of different types of diet on an individual's ability to perform tests of strength, speed, and endurance. The bicycle ergometer can also be used to measure other physical abilities, such as the effects of cigarette smoking on endurance.

bile A yellowish fluid produced by the liver and stored in the gall bladder, from which it is released as needed into the small intestine. Bile contributes to the alkalinity of the digestive tract and helps the emulsification of fats so they can be absorbed from the intestine. It is composed of a number of substances, including bile salts, cholesterol, bilirubin, and electrolytes. Also called *gall*. See *bile salts*.

bile salts Substances contained in bile that help in the digestion of fats. They break up large fat globules into smaller ones, enabling the fats to be broken down further into fatty acids by enzymes in the digestive tract. Bile salts are derived by the body's chemical processes from cholesterol.

biliousness A health condition caused by excessive bile secretion and characterized by nausea, headache, constipation, and general abdominal distress.

binder Any substance added to loosely assembled elements to promote cohesion among the particles. Casein and starch are often used as binders in tablets because they expand easily in water and disintegrate, or dissolve, quickly. Products designed to dissolve slowly may contain a digestible mucilage.

bioaccumulation The accumulation by plants and animals of chemicals, such as pollutants, from the environment. Examples include the bioaccumulation of DDT and other pesticides by fish, birds, and other animals eaten by humans, whose body tissues in turn accumulate the pollutants stored in the fat of the animals consumed as food. Some toxic elements, such as mercury and lead, become stored in human body tissues through bioaccumulation.

bioenergetics A branch of biology concerned with energy relations and changes within a plant or animal.

bioflavonoids A group of widely distributed substances found in plant food sources that apparently play a role in maintaining normal conditions in the walls of blood vessels. The group includes rutin and hesperidin. Bioflavonoid sources include citrus fruits, particularly the area between the pulp and the rind. They are sometimes identified as vitamin P, although there is a lack of evidence that they qualify as true vitamins.

biological value A rating of food proteins with respect to the efficiency with which a given protein supplies the body's nitrogen requirements. The closer a protein can come to furnishing the needed amounts and proportions of the essential amino acids, thereby keeping the body in the proper nitrogen balance for growth or maintenance, the higher is its biological value. Egg protein, which rates the highest with a BV (biological value) of 100, is the standard by which other proteins are measured. See *egg replacement value*.

biosynthesis The process whereby enzymes or other catalysts within living tissues create new substances from chemical compounds or ions present. One example is the biosynthesis of niacin from the amino acid tryptophan in human tissues.

biotin A B-complex vitamin required or produced by all known living organisms. It is abundantly distributed in foods that are sources of other B vitamins. It is also produced by bacteria that normally exist in the digestive tracts of humans and other animals.

    A deficiency of biotin is unusual but it is possible in two rather common situations. One is the presence of sulfa drugs and other antibiotics taken to destroy a bacterial infection in the body; in the process, they may also destroy the bacteria in the intestinal tract that manufacture the bulk of a person's supply of biotin. The second situation can develop from eating raw egg white. Egg white contains a substance known as avidin that combines with biotin to form a complex that cannot be absorbed by the digestive tract. Somewhat ironically, the cure for "egg-white injury" is the administration of egg yolks, which are a rich source of fresh biotin. Biotin binding does not result from eating egg whites that have been cooked.

The importance of maintaining adequate levels of biotin was demonstrated in experimental animals and human volunteers when they were fed diets containing a large proportion of raw egg white. They experienced lesions of the skin and tongue, nausea, anorexia, muscle pain, insomnia, and personality changes dominated by intense depression. Some animals developed paralysis of the hindquarters; most animals with brown or black hair showed premature graying and a peculiar hair loss around the eyes, giving an "eye spectacle" appearance to their features. All the subjects recovered within a few days after receiving doses of biotin. In addition to preventing such defects, biotin is important in synthesizing fatty acids, in the metabolism of glucose, and in the formation of glyocgen, or body starch, and the amino acid, aspartic acid. Also called *vitamin H*.

biscuits A term that in the United States means bakery products manufactured with a nonyeast, chemically leavened dough. In Great Britain and some other countries, biscuits are a nonleavened, flat, crisp, dough product. Biscuit literally means "twice cooked," exposed first to high heat for baking, then to lower heat for drying. Biscuits are sometimes classified as sponge goods, such as yeast-leavened soda crackers; chemically leavened crackers, including graham crackers; and sweet goods, such as fig bars and shortbreads.

bismuth A metallic element used in certain medicines, such as antacids and other preparations designed to treat inflammations of the digestive tract and act as remedies for skin diseases.

bitter almond A peachlike fruit that grows on a small tree found in southern Europe, the Middle East, and parts of the United States. The kernels contain a deadly poison, hydrocyanic acid, which is removed while processing them into an oil used in flavoring beverages, ice creams, candies, bakery products, gelatin desserts, and other foods that may benefit from a potent but mild almond aroma.

blackstrap molasses An industrial grade of molasses that is the final fraction in the process of extracting sucrose from cane or beet sugar. The final fraction represents the residue of the plant syrup beyond which it is not worthwhile to try to extract any more sugar. As a result, blackstrap molasses has a relatively low sugar content for a syrup and is favored by some individuals as a source of calcium, iron, thiamine, and riboflavin.

black tongue A fungus infection that produces a dark, hairlike coating on the surface of the tongue. The condition usually causes no particular symptoms and is treated with antibiotics.

bleaching and maturing agents Substances such as calcium phosphate that are added to freshly milled wheat flour to make it "age" faster. Such agents are usually used as additives because flour millers cannot afford to allow natural, fresh wheat flour, which is yellowish in color, to remain in storage for the several months needed for it to become the mature white powder that can be formed into an elastic dough. Bleaching and maturing agents are prohibited by laws in some countries.

blister A collection of fluid under the skin caused by an irritation of the skin tissues from exposure to heat, pressure, or an irritating chemical. The fluid in a common water blister is lymph that has leaked from the injured cells. When a blood vessel is broken, the fluid beneath the skin may be a mixture of lymph and blood. If the skin over a blister is broken, it should be treated as a wound.

blood The fluid that circulates through the heart, arteries, veins, and capillaries, transporting oxygen from the lungs and nutrients from the digestive system to tissues throughout the body. Blood also transports carbon dioxide from the tissues to the lungs and other metabolic waste products to the kidneys for excretion. It also carries hormones, antibodies, and blood-clotting substances and helps regulate body temperature. Blood is sometimes considered as two parts—the fluid portion, or plasma, which is 92 percent water, 7 percent proteins, and 1 percent inorganic salts; and the solid particles, composed of blood cells and platelets suspended in the fluid.

blood-brain barrier A mechanism of the walls of blood vessels serving the brain and central nervous system that seems to screen substances in the blood, preventing or delaying the transfer of certain substances into cells of nerve tissues. One example is the manner in which the blood-brain barrier screens sugar molecules, permitting glucose to pass into brain cells but preventing other sugars from leaving the blood vessels. The barrier also permits the entry into brain tissues of essential amino acids needed by the brain for the synthesis of other amino acids.

blood cells The erythrocytes (red blood cells) and leukocytes (white blood cells) that constitute the major portion of suspended particles in blood. The red blood cells, of which the average body contains 35 trillion, are concave in shape to provide a large surface area for transporting oxygen. White blood cells lack the hemoglobin of red cells and are colorless. They are larger than red cells but fewer in number and are able to move about like independent organisms. The main function of white cells is to provide the body with a defense against infections. See *hemoglobin; white blood cells.*

blood-cholesterol test A laboratory test for the level of cholesterol in the blood. Although cholesterol is generally associated with heart and circulatory disorders, the blood-cholesterol test is primarily a part of liver function studies since the liver plays a major role in cholesterol metabolism. A blood cholesterol level greatly in excess of 260 mg. of cholesterol per 100 ml. of blood serum may be a sign of liver disease. It may also be a sign of hypothyroidism and several other disorders. The normal range is 135 to 260. Blood cholesterol is measured after a patient has fasted for a given period of time.

blood clotting The formation of a jelly-like mesh of blood cells and other substances in the blood over an area of a blood vessel that has been cut, ruptured, or otherwise damaged. The blood clot begins to form on the damaged wall of the vessel within minutes after an injury occurs as a natural defense against blood loss. Blood clotting requires a series of a dozen steps and is believed to be triggered by blood platelets, microscopic blood cells which disintegrate when they touch a rough edge on an injured blood vessel wall. The main purpose of the clot is to form a temporary patch over a leaking blood vessel. However, a rough surface on a blood vessel wall can also trigger a clot to be formed in an otherwise healthy blood vessel. This can result in a dangerous clot floating through the bloodstream as a thrombus, which might cause a heart attack, stroke, or other damage.

blood count The number of blood cells in a given amount of blood, the amount usually being 1 ml.^{3} The count also specifies whether it represents red or white blood cells or blood platelets. In addition, a differential blood count may report the number of different kinds of white cells in the sample. The normal red blood count (RBC) is between 4.2 and 5.9 million per ml.^{3}; the white blood count (WBC) ranges from 4,800 to 10,800 per ml.^{3}; the platelet count is between 200,000 and 350,000 per ml.^{3}. A cubic millimeter (ml.^{3}) is about the size of a pinhead.

blood lipids The fatty substances circulating in the bloodstream, mainly cholesterol and triglycerides. Both types of fats are carried by four different kinds of fat-protein molecules called *lipoproteins*. They are: (1) chylomicrons, the largest particles, which appear in the blood shortly after eating and mainly carry triglycerides; (2) very low-density lipoproteins (VLDLs), which carry mainly triglycerides and appear in the blood prominently between meals; (3) low-density lipoproteins (LDLs), which carry most of the cholesterol; and (4) high-density lipoproteins (HDLs), which are the smallest particles and carry some cholesterol. High LDL levels seem to be associated with athersoclerosis and an increased risk of coronary heart disease, but many other health factors are also involved, such as heredity.

blood nutrients The food substances essential for the body to produce adequate amounts of normal blood cells. Examples include iron and niacin for the formation of hemoglobin, and vitamin B-12 and folacin for the formation of red blood cells from hemoglobin and other components.

blood plasma The fluid portion of the blood. Plasma accounts for more than half the volume of the blood and is composed of 92 percent water, 7 percent protein, and an assortment of antibodies, inorganic salts, hormones, enzymes, serum albumin, gamma-globulin, and fibrinogen. When fibrinogen, an important blood-clotting factor, is removed from the plasma, the remaining fluid portion is called *serum*.

blood platelets The numerous tiny, round, clear bodies circulating in the bloodstream with the responsibility for starting a blood clot when they find a rough surface on a blood vessel wall. Contact with a rough spot causes a platelet to disintegrate. As they disintegrate, they release a chemical that begins constriction of blood flow in the area and the release of various clotting factors, such as prothrombin. Blood clots also begin accidentally when platelets hit a rough inner surface of a blood vessel that has not been damaged.

blood pressure The pressure of the circulating blood against the walls of the blood vessels, usually the walls of the arteries. Blood pressure is determined by the force of the contractions of the heart in pumping blood; the elasticity of the arteries; the resistance to blood flow by the arterioles, which regulate blood flow to the capillaries; the quantity of blood; and the thickness of the blood. Blood pressure is measured in terms of systolic pressure, produced by contraction of the heart, and diastolic, the pressure recorded during the relaxation period of the heart muscle. It is recorded as systolic/diastolic, as in the example of 125/80. The numbers represent the distance the blood pressure would raise a column of mercury in millimeters.

blood serum The blood plasma from which the fibrinogen has been removed, or the clear liquid that remains after a sample of blood has been allowed to clot completely. See *blood clotting; blood plasma*.

blood sugar The amount of glucose, a basic sugar unit, in the blood. The normal range is between 70 and 100 mg. per 100 ml. of blood, depending on the type of test, since some methods measure substances that react like glucose in addition to "true glucose." If the true glucose level is greater than 120 mg. per 100 ml. of blood, a glucose tolerance test is recommended. Glucose may also be measured in urinalysis tests. In addition to diabetes mellitus, a high blood sugar level may be caused by adrenal, pituitary, or thyroid gland disorders, or to pheochromocytoma, a type of adrenal gland tumor. A blood sugar test is usually based on a sample of blood taken at least 2 hr. after any food intake.

blood types Any of the numerous categories of inherited red blood cells that are identified by the way they react as antigens. Nearly 100 different blood types are known, although the four basic groups, A, B, O, and AB, established in the early twentieth century, are the most important. Also important is the Rh system, which can cause an incompatibility of blood groups between the mother and the fetus. All blood types are related to the body's immune system in which any substance regarded as foreign is rejected by the body's tissues. Thus, when giving a blood transfusion, as in kidney transplant surgery, incompatibility of inherited blood types can result in rejection, usually with tragic results. The A, B, O, AB, and Rh factors have the greatest antigenic activity.

blood urea nitrogen A measure of the amount of nitrogen in the blood of a person. The amount of urea in a person's body increases with the amount of protein in the diet and urea is normally excreted in the urine. When the kidneys fail to function normally, the amount of urea that cannot be excreted accumulates in the blood. An abnormally high level of urea in the blood is a sign of kidney disease. Abbreviated *BUN*.

blood vessels Any of the tubular structures that carry blood to organs and tissues throughout the body, including arteries, veins, arterioles, venules, and capillaries.

BMR See *basal metabolic rate*.

body fat The amount of fat in the body, which can be an indirect measure of the health of the individual. Most of the body's fuel reserves are stored in fat deposits under the skin and around deep organs of the body, as a practical measure by nature since 1 oz. of fat can store as many calories of energy as 2 oz. of pure sugar. The average adult human carries between 24 and 37 lb. of fat, or between 15 and 25 percent of total body weight. As a person ages, fat gradually replaces muscle tissue—even if body weight does not increase. Thus, a person whose adult body weight increases by 25 percent in effect doubles the original 25 percent of body fat.

body regulators A term sometimes applied to nutrients other than carbohydrates, proteins, and fats that help regulate the body by assisting in metabolism and other physiological processes. Body regulators include water, vitamins, and minerals.

body temperature The normal temperature of the body, which for humans is usually considered to be 98.6°F or 37°C when measured in the mouth with a clinical or fever thermometer. When measured rectally, the figures are 99.2°F and 37.3°C. These figures are averages for normal persons and individual temperatures may vary between morning and night, before or after a meal, or as a result of exercise or excitement. An oral temperature reading of 100°F or 37.8°C, or higher, is considered a fever. A temperature below 96°F or 35.6°C is a sign of hypothermia or collapse. See *temperature regulation*.

body types The different kinds of more or less natural body builds seen in different individuals. One system of classifying body types recognizes a soft, rounded build, called *endomorph*; a strong, muscular-appearing build, known as *mesomorph*; and the delicate, thin, flat-chested type, identified as *ectomorph*. Some efforts have been made to find associations between body build types and personality types, but the subject remains quite controversial even after hundreds of years of study.

body weight The weight of a person's body. The figures vary considerably because of height, age, and body build. Average or so-called normal weights are based on studies of very large populations, such as weights of young men drafted for military service or women applying for insurance policies, and are adjusted periodically to match changes in the populations measured. A young person today, for example, is likely to be somewhat taller and heavier than his or her parents or grandparents at the same age. See the height-weight table on page 228.

bomb calorimeter A device used to measure the number of calories in a sample of food. It consists of a container in which the food sample can be sealed with a quantity of pure oxygen and a water bath in which the food container can be submerged. After the container is submerged, the contents are ignited by an electric circuit. A thermometer in the water bath measures the temperature change in the water. By knowing the amount of water and its temperature at the beginning and end of the food combustion, one can determine the amount of heat in calories produced by burning a measured amount of food. By this technique, nutrition experts can tell, for example, that a fresh egg weighing 50 g. (slightly less than 2 oz.) yields 78 calories of energy.

bone The rigid structural material of the bodies of vertebrates, composed mainly of calcium compounds, and generally organized in movable segments that form the skeleton.

The number of bones in the human body is 270 at birth but only 206 in adulthood because a number of the separate bones fuse during growth. For example, nine vertebrae present at birth fuse into two vertebrae, the sacrum and coccyx, later in life. Because the bones are on the inside of the body, humans and other vertebrate animals can grow faster than species whose protective structure is outside the body, as in the case of shellfish.

Some bones, such as those that form the skull, are relatively flat. Long bones, like those of the arms and legs, are generally tubular, a natural design that gives maximum strength with a minimum amount of material. Bone generally has the strength of cast iron, an important feature of the skeleton since the body weight on a leg bone may be equivalent to 1,200 lb. per square inch.

However, bone is not simply inert material, like iron or concrete. It is composed of dynamic, living tissue. About one-third of living bone material is organic tissue similar to that found in the skin and tendons; 20 percent of the weight of living bone is water. The remainder is a matrix of mineral salts, including nearly all of the body's supply of calcium, plus phosphorus, magnesium, and other elements. Living bone contains blood vessels, nerves, and a variety of cells, including *osteoblasts*, which build new bone material and repair damaged bone tissues; *osteocytes*, which maintain the bone material surrounding them with nutrients taken from the passing blood flow; and *osteoclasts*, which dissolve bone from areas where it is no longer required so the minerals can be used elsewhere.

bone marrow The soft, spongelike material in the cavities of bones. Bone marrow is sometimes classified as red marrow and yellow marrow. Red marrow, found in the skull, breastbone, and ribs, is the part of the body where blood cells—red and white blood cells and platelets—are produced. Yellow marrow, located mainly in the long bones, is primarily fatty tissue and has no blood-producing role. As one grows older, much of the red marrow turns to yellow marrow. However, in an emergency such as a hemorrhage, yellow marrow can be converted to red marrow to increase production of blood cells.

bone meal A meal made from cattle bones, which are ground or pulverized, available as a source of calcium and other nutrients for persons who avoid milk because of allergies or adherence to a vegan diet. Bone meal usually contains some magnesium, phosphorus, and other minerals, such as copper, fluorine, and nickel. Because of rules that permit ground meats sold in retail stores to contain ground bone, most Americans have been consuming bone meal with their hamburgers. Two average bone meal tablets contain approximately the same amount of calcium as 1 cup of whole milk.

borborygmus A fancy medical term for the rumbling noises made by gas moving through the intestines. It may be pronounced as *bor-bo-rig-mus*, in the event one needs to explain the sound in polite company.

boron A mineral necessary for normal plant growth and found in the human body in trace amounts. However, numerous experiments have failed to establish a nutritional need for boron in animals.

bottled water See *distilled water; mineral water.*

botulism A very serious type of food poisoning caused by the presence in food of a neurotoxin, or nerve poison, excreted by a bacteria that lives without oxygen.
 Botulism is particularly unusual among food poison situations in that it does not cause the stomach upsets normally associated with food poisoning. Instead, it may produce symptoms as much as 18 hours to 8 days later that begin with eye problems, such as double vision or sudden difficulty in focusing the eyes. The visual disturbances may be accompanied by fatigue and weakness, with difficulty in swallowing.
 These disorders may be difficult for a doctor to diagnose because the person may appear normal except for the effects caused by the toxin, which blocks the normal transmission of certain nerve impulses. In most cases, the food containing the neurotoxin has been consumed or discarded so it is not available for testing, making the physician's task even more difficult. Unless emergency treatment is administered, death usually occurs within a few days from paralysis of the respiratory system.
 Botulism food poisoning occurs most commonly from eating improperly canned or otherwise preserved foods in which the bacterial spores have had an opportunity to secrete their poison. Foods most often involved are string beans, corn, mushrooms, olives, beets, spinach, asparagus, seafood, pork, and beef. Improperly smoked fish can also be a source of botulism. The toxin, which may remain after the bacteria have been killed, is destroyed by cooking for at least 30 min. at temperatures above 175°F or 80°C. Although 90 percent of botulism cases result from eating home-canned foods, the toxin may also occur in commercially prepared foods. If any canned or otherwise preserved food has a strange odor or is in a bulging or damaged container, it should be discarded. Food that shows signs of contamination should *never* be tasted.

bran The tough outer layer of cereal grains, such as wheat or rice. It is composed mostly of indigestible cellulose, but also contains carbohydrates and some vitamins and minerals. The cellulose content of bran provides bulk, or roughage, to the diet, just as the cellulose in salad vegetables provides bulk, which aids in digestion. Bran products sold as breakfast cereals and bakery products are usually combined with a milled grain, such as wheat flour, which makes them more palatable and nourishing.

breath-holding test A physical fitness test of the cardiovascular system and lung capacity. The test requires the person to step on and off a bench approximately 15 in. high repeatedly for a period of 1 min. At the end of the minute, the person must hold his breath for as long as possible. If the individual is unable to hold the breath for at least 30 sec., it is considered a sign that the heart-lung systems are inadequate.

brewer's yeast A microscopic one-celled type of fungus used commercially to ferment sugars to alcohol and also as a dietary supplement because of its unique concentration of B vitamins and amino acids. Brewer's yeast was used as a medicine more than 3,500 years ago in Egypt, but only recently have medical scientists become aware of its therapeutic value in treating a variety of physical and mental disorders, particularly pellagra. A serving of brewer's yeast can provide 18 amino acids, 11 vitamins, and 14 minerals in varying amounts. See *baker's yeast; yeast*.

brine A strong salt solution used in pickling and preserving foods. Sea water is a natural form of brine. It is usually a source of sodium chloride, plus bromine, iodine, and potassium compounds. Brine is also used in food processing as a freezing mixture since a solution containing 23 percent sodium chloride enables foods to be kept at temperatures as low as $-21°C$ or $-6°F$; however, the brine mixture is not used to freeze unpackaged foods because it would give the food an unpalatable salty flavor.

British Dietary Standards The daily intake of nutrients recommended as sufficient or greater for all persons living in the United Kingdom. The British standards generally recommend more total calories and protein than U.S. standards, but smaller amounts of certain vitamins. More than a dozen other countries, including Canada, have their own scale of recommended daily nutrient intakes.

bromelin An enzyme obtained from pineapples that is used as an additive to tenderize meat. Also called *bromelain*.

brominated vegetable oil A vegetable oil to which bromine has been added to make the oil equivalent in density to water. Brominated vegetable oils carry flavorings that can be dispersed through soft drinks without rising to the top of the beverage, the densities being approximately equal. The dispersed vegetable oil is also used to give the soft drink an appearance of body because it produces a cloudy effect which suggests thickness and richness. Brominated vegetable oils are prohibited in some countries because of evidence of associations with adverse health effects in laboratory animals. Abbreviated *BVO*. See *soft drinks*.

bromine An element that is widely distributed in nature, particularly in sea water, and is a chemical cousin of chlorine and fluorine. Bromine is used in numerous medications, antiseptics, and deodorants. The average human body contains about 3 parts per million of bromine. Large amounts are toxic.

brown fat A type of fat found in varying amounts in the newborn and sometimes in adults in the neck and shoulder region. It is brown in color, as distinguished *browning*

from the usual white or yellowish color of fat deposits. Brown fat also differs from regular fat in the way it releases energy when metabolized. It contains nerve cells and mitochondria, which rapidly mobilize the fat for heat production in response to cold stimuli, but it is not influenced by starvation like white fat.

browning   A term used to describe the color changes that occur in some cut fruits and vegetables because of the action of enzymes present. Browning also occurs in foods from other causes, such as the carmelization of sugars when heated. Coffee beans, for example, are grayish- to bluish-green before they are roasted; the brown color is caused by carmelizing the carbohydrates. Browning may result in adverse color effects that make foods less appetizing, but in many cases browning is acceptable. Brown beer, dark molasses, brown bread, and the browning of grapes to produce raisins often increases the acceptability of these foods.

brown sugar   See *sugar*.

brucellosis   An infectious disease caused by a bacteria family that affects goats, cattle, and pigs. It can be transmitted to humans through infected milk or contact with the carcass of a diseased animal. Symptoms include fever, headaches, and anemia. It is also known as *undulant fever* because the main symptom is a fever that fluctuates widely in temperature range. Humans who drink milk can avoid the disease by consuming only milk that has been pasteurized.

BSP test   A shortened name for the bromsulphalein retention test of liver function. Bromsulphalein is a dye that can be injected into the bloodstream. A blood sample taken 45 min. later indicates the percentage of the dye absorbed by the liver. If the liver is normal, all the dye will be absorbed and excreted through the bile duct. If liver disease is present, more than 10 percent of the dye will remain in the blood. The test is not used when the patient has a jaundice condition, another sign of liver malfunction. Also called *sulfobromopthalein test*.

buffer   A substance that helps maintain the acid-base balance in the body by counteracting any change in the amount of acidity or alkalinity of the blood or other tissues. The buffer itself is either a weak acid or weak alkaline substance, such as carbonic acid or sodium bicarbonate. Proteins, phosphates, and hemoglobin also play buffering roles as needed. The lungs and kidneys, by regulating levels of sodium and carbon dioxide in the body, continually adjust the amount of carbonic acid or sodium bicarbonate needed to buffer the blood.

building blocks A term sometimes used to describe the role of subunits of nutrients, such as the amino acids that are the building blocks of proteins or the glucose units that are linked together in complex sugar molecules. See *amino acid*.

bulimia An abnormally excessive appetite. An injury to the hypothalamus, such as a tumor growth, can produce this disorder. It has also been associated with some cases of anorexia nervosa. When the cause is psychogenic, a binge of extreme overeating is usually followed by forced vomiting. This practice can result in a serious loss of essential nutrients.

bulk The fiber foods, such as fruits, vegetables, and cereal brans, that contain cellulose. The cellulose components serve primarily as structural and protective parts of plant foods and cannot be digested by humans, who lack the enzymes needed to break cellulose down into easily absorbed carbohydrate units. However, bulk is helpful and usually important for normal digestive tract function because it enters into the formation and movement of feces through the intestine. In addition to cellulose, substances known as hemicellulose, lignin, gums, pectins, and pentosans provide bulk. Also called *roughage*. See *fiber*.

butterfat The total crude fatty material removed from whole milk. The amount of butterfat per volume of milk varies between 2 and 8 percent and is determined by adding an acid to a sample of milk to remove the protein part of the mixture, then whirling the remainder in a centrifuge to force the fatty portion to the top of the container. The total amount of fatty substances separated in this manner is regarded as butterfat. In most countries butter is required to contain at least 80 percent butterfat by weight. Ice creams contain between 10 and 20 percent butterfat. Also called *milkfat*.

buttermilk A milk product that is similar to skim milk except that it contains lactic acid. Buttermilk is manufactured in two forms. One, the original method, involves simply collecting the fluid by-product resulting from the churning of cream into butter. The second, called *cultured buttermilk*, is produced by adding lactic acid bacteria to skim milk. Cultured buttermilk contains approximately 9 times as much lactic acid as regular buttermilk. A cultured buttermilk is also likely to have a more acidic flavor than regular buttermilk made from sweet cream.

butyric acid A fatty acid found in butter and certain other food fats, including the fatty portion of whole milk. When butter becomes rancid, the unpleasant aroma is produced by the release of butyric acid from the butterfat complex.

by-product A substance or object produced as a result of a process that is primarily intended to yield a different substance or object. Examples include the production of wheat germ and wheat bran as by-products of the primary function of milling wheat in order to obtain white flour.

C

cadmium A mineral that accumulates in the body and is important mainly because of the adverse health effects associated with it. It is poorly absorbed from substances in the diet but the average adult body contains levels of about 7 parts per 10-million, the proportion increasing with age. Some experts believe cadmium may have an effect on blood pressure. It is known to be carcinogenic and to cause anemia by interfering with copper and iron metabolism. Cadmium enters the food supply through processing and packaging methods and by irrigation of food crops with water contaminated by mining and smelting industries. Cadmium poisoning by eating rice irrigated with polluted water has occurred in Japan.

café coronary A popular term for a choking episode that is caused by a piece of food that obstructs the trachea, the tube leading from the throat to the lungs. The term derived its name from an early belief that people who suddenly turned speechless and collapsed while eating had suffered a heart attack. Recent investigation found the symptoms were caused by an inability to breathe or talk because of food obstruction in the trachea which, if not treated, can lead to death within a few minutes. See *Heimlich maneuver*.

caffeine A central nervous system stimulant that occurs naturally in a wide variety of plant products, including coffee, tea, cola, cocoa, maté, and guarana. The amount of caffeine varies from about 1 percent of the dry weight of mild, Arabica-type coffee beans to more than 4 percent in Java black teas. However, the proportions change with beverage use. For example, tea contains more caffeine than coffee but a smaller amount is used in preparing the beverage so that a cup of brewed coffee may contain twice as much caffeine as a cup of brewed tea. A fatal dose of caffeine is about 10 gr., the amount in about 100 cups of regular coffee.

calciferol A crystalline from of *ergocalciferol*. See this entry; *vitamin D*.

calcification The accumulation of calcium salts in soft tissues of the body, causing them to become hard and stiff. Calcium deposits are commonly in the form of calcium carbonate or calcium phosphate. The term may also be applied to describe the deposition of calcium compounds in the formation of bone. Arteriosclerosis, or hardening of the arteries due to calcium deposits, is sometimes called *Moenckeberg's calcification.* In other organs, such as the stomach, calcification may be caused by acid conditions that cause calcium to precipitate from body fluids.

calcium A chemical element that is the most abundant mineral in the human body. Almost all of the body's calcium is combined with phosphorus, as calcium phosphate, in the skeleton and teeth. Only about 1 percent of the body calcium is in the blood, extracellular, and soft tissues of the human organism. Calcium is vitally involved in a number of physiological processes, including the coagulation of blood, maintenance of cell membranes, the transmission of nerve impulses, hormone secretion, enzyme reactions, and neuromuscular activities.

The average human adult body contains about 1.1 kg., or slightly less than 2.5 lb. of calcium, part of which is moving constantly into or out of the bones. The bones, far from being inactive, like stone, are very dynamic organs that undergo continuous changes to meet the varying calcium needs of the individual. They also serve as a calcium reservoir for molecules of the mineral needed for normal body activities, such as muscle contractions. The calcium levels of various body systems are regulated by the parathyroid glands. When the level of calcium in the blood drops below a particular level, the parathyroid glands trigger a mechanism that scrapes a bit of calcium from the skeleton for use in nerves, muscles, and other body parts. When there is more than enough calcium in the blood, the parathyroid glands are automatically turned off. A high blood level of calcium may also result in excretion of the excess.

The average adult requirement for calcium amounts to around 10 mg. (1 mg. equals 1/30,000 of 1 oz.) per kilogram of body weight. The average woman, therefore, needs about 10 times 60 (kg.), or 600 mg., of calcium and the average man about 700 mg. Actual daily adult calcium intake has been found to range from as low as 200 mg. to more than 2,000 mg. per day, with the average in the United States hovering around 600 mg.

The actual amount of calcium available to the human body from the diet depends on a wide range of factors, such as age, the amount of vitamin D, lactose, growth hormone, and several amino acids. About 75 percent of the calcium in a child's diet may be absorbed, whereas the figure drops to about 30 percent in later years. Vitamin D, growth hormone, lactose, and certain amino acids help increase absorption. But certain synthetic hormones, excess fatty acids in the intestine, indigestible substances in bran, and foods that contain calcium-binding chemicals, such as oxalic acid, can reduce the amount of the mineral absorbed from the diet. In addition to calcium lost through excretion of feces and urine, a substantial amount—as much as 1,000 mg. per day—can be lost in sweat by persons working hard in high temperatures.

Milk is the most convenient source of calcium for most people. An average serving provides about 285 mg. of calcium. But on a per-weight basis, a 100-g. (about 3 oz.) serving of cheddar cheese provides 750 mg. of calcium, compared to 118 mg. for an equal weight of milk. Molasses, ice cream, dried figs, and cooked leafy vegetables also provide more calcium per 100-g. serving than milk. Runners-up include broccoli, bread, cottage cheese, peanut butter, and pitted dates. One of the poorest sources of calcium is cooked whole-grain cereal—before the cream is added to bring the average up sharply.

A calcium deficiency results in a softening of the bones and teeth, a condition known as *rickets* when it involves children. A similar disorder that can develop in adults, *osteomalacia*, is one in which the bones become fragile and break easily. *Osteoporosis*, a disease of older people, characterized by the atrophy of skeletal tissue, is associated with a negative calcium balance in younger years. Other effects include impaired blood clotting and nervous and muscular disorders. When a parathyroid deficiency is involved in low blood calcium levels a condition of convulsive muscle cramps, called *tetany*, can occur.

calcium balance A term used to indicate that a person's intake of calcium is equal to the amount lost by excretion. The term is sometimes modified to indicate what actually is an imbalance. A *negative balance* means that calcium intake is less than the amount lost, while a *positive calcium balance* is another way of saying that intake of calcium exceeds the amount of the mineral lost from the body.

calcium lactate A soluble salt of calcium used to help maintain normal breathing in persons who suffer from a severe form of calcium deficiency. Impaired breathing is a symptom of a complex of medical problems, called *tetany*, that can result from a major calcium imbalance. Because of the role of calcium in supporting normal neuromuscular function, a lack of calcium can cause a wide range of muscle tone spasms, including the muscles that control breathing.

calcium-phosphorus ratio The proportions of calcium and phosphorus recommended for the daily diet to maintain a proper calcium balance. The ratio is approximately 2:3 (calcium:phosphorus). When phosphorus intake greatly exceeds the ratio, calcium may be excreted faster than it is taken into the body, resulting in a negative calcium balance. The ratio is often upset by excessive consumption of soft drinks containing phosphoric acid, a source of phosphorus, plus eating phosphorus-rich meat, fish, eggs, and nuts.

calcium supplement A form of calcium taken in tablet or pill form to supplement the calcium in the person's diet, which may be inadequate for various reasons, for example, a medical problem like osteoporosis. The calcium is consumed in tablets of calcium carbonate, calcium gluconate, or calcium *calculated nutrient content*

lactate, or a combination of calcium compounds. Calcium supplements may also be recommended for pregnant or nursing women.

calculated nutrient content   The protein, fat, carbohydrate, vitamins, or other nutrients in a diet or recipe calculated from food composition tables, and not from direct analysis of the specific foods.

caloric balance   The balance between the calories consumed and the number of calories burned during the same day, week, or other period in work and exercise. If your food intake exceeds your caloric expenditure by more than 100 calories per day, your weight could increase at a rate of 1 lb. per month.

caloric excess   An intake of calories exceeding that required for growth, metabolic processes, and for adult maintenance of desirable weight. Also called *overnutrition*.

caloric modification   Alteration of caloric amounts in a diet according to specific needs. The source may also be varied, such as the proportion taken from fats and carbohydrates.

caloric test   A test that has nothing to do with calories or food but is designed to determine the ability of a person to maintain his sense of balance. A doctor pours warm or cool water into the external ear canal and measures the time it takes for symptoms of dizziness to begin and the time required to recover from the dizzy spell. Because the sense of balance, or equilibrium, is in the ear, the temperature difference between the water and body temperature disturbs the sense of balance and produces the dizzy effects.

calorie   A standard measure of heat. Technically, 1 calorie is the amount of heat required to raise the temperature of 1 kg. of water by 1°C or 1 lb. of water by 4°F.

Because heat is released in the metabolism of food, or in the burning of the same food in a laboratory caloric "bomb," food items are often measured by the amount of calories contained in 1 lb., one serving, or some other unit. The caloric measures of foods generally can be translated in terms of 4 calories per gram of pure carbohydrate, such as sugar, 4 calories per gram of pure protein, and 9 calories per gram of pure fat. The calorie content of 1 g. of alcohol is sometimes included at 7 calories since alcoholic beverages are a source of calories and little else. The numbers of calories per type of food, such as 9 calories per gram of fat, are rounded-off averages. Different kinds of fatty acids may yield slightly different amount of calories. But for practical purposes, the average number is used in calculating the number of calories in a food item or in an entire meal. One pound of fat is equivalent to about 3,500 calories and the average adult body contains an amount of fat equal to approximately 125,000 calories.

The human body requires varying amounts of calories per day for normal daily life functions. The brain, for example, uses about 500 calories per day. To determine the number of calories your own body needs each day, multiply your weight in kilograms (1 kg. equals 2.2 lb.) by 25 if you spend most of your time in bed; by 30 to 35 if you do light office work or housework; 35 to 40 if you are moderately active; and by 40 to 45 if you are a construction worker, farmer, or engaged in a similar job that requires heavy exercise. See *gram calorie; kilocalorie.*

calorie conversion factors Factors used for the conversion of grams of protein, fat, and carbohydrate to kilocalories. The numbers may differ for the same nutrient depending on the source of values, which could be one used primarily in the United States, Europe, or internationally. Calories may also be converted to joules; 1 kilocalorie is equivalent to 4,185.5 joules.

calorie tables The published data used in this and other reference books as general guidelines for the caloric content of various foods. These figures are estimates, usually based on averages of data obtained from laboratory studies by the government or other agencies. It is difficult and usually impractical to be precise about the number of calories in 1 lb. or serving or any other measure of an amount of food because measures are seldom exact. Also, the precise amount of nutrients varies considerably, so that two tomatoes from the same vine or two cows from the same herd are not likely to yield the same amount of vitamins, minerals, or calories per ounce of edible food.

calorimetry The process or technique of measuring heat loss or expenditure. Calorimetry of a human body can be measured by the direct method of immersing the body in a tank of water and measuring the temperature change in the water caused by body heat. An indirect method is to measure the amount of oxygen consumed by a person and the amount of carbon dioxide exhaled during a given period; multiplying the liters of oxygen consumed by a factor of 4.8 gives the approximate number of calories used. The device for either direct or indirect calorimetry is called a *calorimeter.*

Canadian Dietary Standards The recommended daily allowances of nutrients established by the Canadian Council on Nutrition. The figures are approximately the same as those used in the United States except that allowances for vitamins A, B-1, and C are somewhat lower and less iron is recommended for men.

cancer A general term for a large number of different diseases that have in common a wild, uncontrolled growth of new cells which invade and destroy surrounding tissues that were normal. Cancer cells frequently appear as a tumor, or abnormal growth, of tissue. A cancer can migrate from its original source to another part of the body by releasing a few cells into the blood or lymph system to be carried some distance to a different kind of organ. A breast cancer, for example, may be the original source of cancer cells in the lungs and lung cancer can be an original source of cancer of the bone, and so on. See *carcinogenic*.

cancer and diet   The association between a high risk of cancer and the consumption of certain foods, particularly fatty and salted, pickled, and smoked meats, as reported in 1982 by a special panel of the U.S. National Academy of Sciences. The panel, convened at the request of the National Cancer Institute, made its report after a 2-year review of all the recent scientific research into possible food carcinogens.

In addition to finding links between cancer and the consumption of foods high in any kinds of fats, saturated or unsaturated, such as meat, poultry, whole-milk dairy products, and cooking oils, the scientists indicated that certain fruits and vegetables in the diet might have a protective effect against cancer. These include foods rich in vitamin C and beta-carotene, a yellow pigment in plant food sources that can be converted to vitamin A in the body. Foods rich in vitamin C include citrus fruits, tomatoes, and peppers. Foods with a high content of beta-carotene include dark-green leafy vegetables and deep-yellow fruits and vegetables, such as carrots, spinach, and broccoli. Vitamin A and the pro-carotene vitamins are believed to reduce the risk of bladder, breast, lung, and skin cancers. Vitamin-C–rich foods are associated with a lower risk of cancers of the stomach and esophagus. Vegetables of the cabbage family, including broccoli, cauliflower, brussels sprouts, and kale, were found to possess substances that seem to prevent or inhibit cancers.

Smoked sausages, smoked fish, bacon, ham, frankfurters, and bologna were singled out as particularly high in the potentially carcinogenic categories because they are generally fatty meats as well as being cured. Cancer of the stomach is relatively common among people who eat large amounts of such cured meats.

canker sore   See *aphthous ulcer*.

capsules   Small, oval-shaped containers made of gelatin for powders or liquids to be taken by mouth. The gelatin may vary in hardness according to the amount of glycerin used in the gelatin. Generally, powders are packaged in hard capsules and liquids in soft capsules. The gelatin may also be treated with a substance to prevent its disintegration in the stomach, if there is a reason for the capsule to be carried farther along the digestive tract. Capsules vary in size but an average hard capsule contains about 0.5 g. of powder. The smallest capsules are sometimes called *perles*.

carbenoxolone   A substance in licorice root used as a protective agent against excessive gastric juice in the digestive tract. Also called *carbenoxalone*.

carbohydrate loading A dietary practice used by some athletes in activities requiring endurance, particularly marathon running. A low-carbohydrate diet is eaten for several days to deplete the muscles of stored carbohydrates or glycogen. This is followed by ingestion of a carbohydrate-rich diet, one that will overload the muscles' glycogen stores, during the next 3 days before an athletic event.

carbohydrate modification Changes in type or amount of carbohydrates in a therapeutic diet.

carbohydrates A general term for a large group of sugars, starches, and celluloses. Carbohydrates are composed of carbon, hydrogen, and oxygen, generally arranged in the same proportions of those elements regardless of the size, structure, or name of the substance. They are formed in plants by the process of photosynthesis, in which energy from the sun is captured by chlorophyll, the green coloring matter in plants, and used to combine carbon dioxide and water in the environment into sugar molecules. Carbon dioxide and water provide the carbon, hydrogen, and oxygen for the carbohydrates. When carbohydrates are "burned" as energy to move muscles or to provide body warmth, the energy taken from the sun is released and the carbohydrate is changed back into the original carbon dioxide and water molecules. Because carbohydrates are completely biodegradable, they represent an ultimate type of pollution-free fuel.

Carbohydrates are the most abundant source of food in the world, and in most cases, the least expensive type of food. The proportion of carbohydrates in daily meals varies considerably throughout the world. In tropical Third World countries, carbohydrates represent a major part of the diet. At the other extreme are the polar Eskimo cultures which subsist on diets containing little, if any, of the fruits and vegetables that are a prime source of carbohydrates. In most of North America, carbohydrates account for approximately one-half of daily caloric intake.

Both animals and plants depend on carbohydrates as an immediate source of energy. Most people are aware of the quick burst of energy that follows the eating of a candy bar or a similar source of sugar. For animals, humans in particular, carbohydrates are a protein-sparing food, which means that when a person's caloric intake is severly restricted, as during starvation or certain fad diets, the body begins to digest its own tissues for the energy in amino acid molecules; by splitting off the nitrogen-containing portion of amino acids, they can be converted to carbohydrates for use as body fuel. In providing enough carbohydrates, or fats, in the diet, a person can prevent the self-digestion of his own muscles and other body tissues. Carbohydrates are also needed by the body in order to use fats effectively; when carbohydrate metabolism is disrupted, as in diabetes mellitus, metabolism of fats can increase to a rate that is greater than the ability of the body to dispose of its waste products, resulting in ketosis, acidosis, and life-threatening coma.

The human brain is a primary consumer of carbohydrates in the form of the simple sugar, glucose. The brain utilizes glucose at a rate of between 100 and 150 g., or the equivalent of 3 to 5 oz. of pure sugar, per day. That amount is also equivalent to the amount of carbohydrate stored in the liver and other body tissues. Thus, the carbohydrate reserves of the body can be depleted in less than 24 hr. of starvation, after which fat deposits are converted to fuel to keep the individual alive. The blood contains some glucose, or blood sugar, but only enough to fuel the body for about 1 hr. A small amount of carbohydrates, in the form of glycogen, or body starch, are stored in muscle tissue, but again, only enough to sustain the body for a brief period before it is necessary for the metabolic mechanisms to start consuming fats or proteins as carbohydrate substitutes.

Food scientists often divide carbohydrates into two groups identified as *simple sugars* and *compound sugars*. The simple sugars are also divided into *pentoses*, if they have five carbon atoms, and *hexoses*, if they have six carbon atoms. They may also be identified as *monosaccharides*. A compound sugar is composed of two or more molecules of simple sugars. The monosaccharides, such as glucose and fructose, and the *disaccharides*, including maltose, lactose, and sucrose, generally have a sweet taste and dissolve easily in water. Most compound sugars are tasteless, are sometimes difficult to digest, and may not dissolve in water.

Glucose is the basic simple sugar used by the human body as a source of energy. Most complex carbohydrates, with the exception of celluloses, can be converted by the body's chemical factories into simple glucose molecules, just as the body can convert fats and proteins to glucose molecules. Glucose occurs naturally in most fruits and vegetables and is also present, mixed with fructose, in honey. Foods that have a high sugar content, meaning two-thirds or more of their weight is in pure sugars, include beet and cane sugars, honey, syrups, candies, cakes, jams, jellies, preserves, dried apricots, dates, figs, prunes, and raisins. Most fresh fruits have a sugar content of between 10 and 25 percent.

Most grain products, such as cereals, and vegetables contain carbohydrates in the form of starches. A starch molecule is generally composed of a large number of glucose units, usually averaging around 350 simple sugar molecules. Most starches occur in the form of *amylose*, a relatively small chain of glucose molecules, and *amylopectin*, which is a huge complex of thousands of glucose units extending in numerous branches from a long chain. But even the largest starch molecules appear to the naked eye as tiny granules. The proportions of amylose and amylopectin vary in different foods: corn starch is about 20 percent amylose while the starch in wrinkled peas is 70 percent amylose.

Cereal grains, such as wheat, corn, rice, rye, and barley, are rich sources of starch. They may contain as much as 85 percent starch when processed as dry breakfast cereals, crackers, or breads; when prepared as cooked cereals the proportions are lower because of the higher water content. Macaroni, spaghetti, cooked rice, and sweet potatoes are approximately 25 to 35 percent starch, and boiled or baked white potatoes contain about 20 percent starch. Starch in raw foods occurs in granules concealed in cellulose capsules and is indigestible until the cellulose seal is broken to make the starch accessible to digestive enzymes in the body. Milling and cooking foods breaks the cellulose barrier.

Both amylose and amylopectin starches break down easily when exposed to the digestive enzymes, such as pytalin in the human saliva glands. Amylase splits into maltose and glucose while amylopectin breaks into maltose, glucose, and dextrin units. Further digestive processes reduce the subunits into simple glucose molecules. Cellulose is composed of numerous building blocks of glucose, but humans lack the enzymes to digest the carbohydrate material that comprises most of the structural parts of fruits and vegetables. However, cellulose is an important part of the diet because it provides the bulk necessary for normal elimination of other waste products of the digestive tract.

carbon An element that occurs in nature both as an uncombined substance, as in coal, and in a vast number of combinations essential to life processes. Although carbon has a black color in coal and graphite, it can also be colorless or white when it occurs in diamonds. Carbon is found combined with oxygen in both carbon monoxide and carbon dioxide and as soda water in the form of carbonic acid. Salts of carbonic acid are called *carbonates*, which are components of dolomite and a form of iron used to treat anemia.

carboxyl groups Chemical units that occur frequently in foods and tissues of living organisms and consist of a carbon atom separated from a hydrogen atom by two oxygen atoms, as in the formula COOH. One example is acetic acid, which is CH_3COOH. Many metabolic activities involve the manipulation of carboxyl groups in various food molecules.

carcinogenic A term applied to substances or processes that can cause the development of cancer cells in living tissue. A number of chemicals, such as benzene and nitrosamines, have been found to be carcinogenic in laboratory animals. Sunlight and x-rays are also capable of producing cancer cells by disrupting the normal metabolic activity of cells in living tissue. Hormones, such as diethylstilbesterol, viruses, gallstones, and aflatoxin molds on peanuts are other examples of carcinogenic factors. U.S. Food and Drug Administration regulations prohibit the use of any known carcinogen in any food products sold for human consumption. The rule has been extended to cover natural foods, like saffrole, that are considered carcinogenic. However, the laws do not cover

cardiovascular disease Any disease that affects the heart and circulatory system, such as *atherosclerosis*. See this entry.

cardiovascular fitness The ability of the heart and circulatory system to transport oxygen from the lungs to the tissue cells throughout the body.

caries The death or decay of bone material. The term is commonly used to identify the disease caused in teeth when microorganisms in the mouth metabolize carbohydrates, producing a waste product that erodes tooth material. Caries can also develop from other causes in other types of bone, such as spinal caries caused by the action of tuberculosis bacteria on the vertebrae and the cartilage disks that separate them. Caries is derived from a Latin word that literally means "rottenness." Although caries and cavities are sometimes used interchangeably, it should be remembered that caries is the name of a disease and cavities are the result of the disease.

carnitine A substance that is a vitamin for insects, particularly mealworms, but not for humans. However, carnitine is a vital substance for normal human health because it enables the heart muscle to burn fatty acids, a prime source of fuel for the heart. An absence of carnitine can be a cause of heart disorders, but a normal human manufactures his own supply. Dietary sources include meats, fish, and yeast. Because of its role as a vitamin for insects, particularly a species with the Latin name *tenebrio*, carnitine is sometimes identified as vitamin B-t.

carotenes A group of carotenoid plant pigments that contribute to the yellow and orange colors of certain fruits and vegetables, such as carrots. These pigments are called carotenes because they were first extracted from carrots in 1831. There are three basic types of carotene, identified by the Greek letters alpha, beta, and gamma. *Beta-carotene*, found in most common yellow fruits and vegetables, is important to human health because the body can easily convert it to vitamin A. Other types of carotene can also be converted to vitamin A, but larger amounts of these carotenes are required to produce the same amount of the vitamin.

carotenoids The name of a group of pigments, including the carotenes, that give color to a wide variety of fruits and vegetables, including peaches, tomatoes, squash, peppers, and even banana skins. In addition to the carotenes, the carotenoids include *lycopene*, which is the reddish pigment of tomatoes, watermelons, and rose hips, and *crocetin*, which helps give saffron its yellowish-orange coloration. See *carotenes*.

carrageenan A substance obtained from Irish moss, a type of algae or seaweed, and used in foods like puddings and pie fillings because of its ability to form a weak type of gelatin with the proteins in milk. It is used in chocolate milk to prevent the chocolate from settling out of the milk and in evaporated milk to prevent the separation of the butterfat portion. Irish moss, which is actually the name applied to a number of different seaweeds, grows mainly in the Atlantic Ocean, from North America to Europe and North Africa. Carrageenan is extracted from the seaweed with boiling water. Also called *carrageenin; carragheen.*

cartilage An elastic, semihard tissue, commonly known as gristle, that forms parts of the features of the head, such as the external ears and nose. In the human embryo, the patterns for most of the bones are formed first as cartilage, then gradually replaced by mineral salts and other bone material.

casein The name applied to milk proteins. Casein is not a single protein, but a substance composed of a number of different proteins that have somewhat different properties. The main component is a type of alpha-casein made of 199 amino acids linked together in a long daisy chain. Casein contains all the essential amino acids and many of the nonessential amino acids.

catabolism The phase of metabolism in which nutrient materials are broken down into simpler chemical units that may be consumed as body fuel or used as building blocks for other molecules needed by the body. Catabolism is the opposite of *anabolism*, which is the body's use of nutrient units to build or maintain tissue structures and functions.

catalase An enzyme found in plant and animal tissues, including human cells, with the function of neutralizing hydrogen peroxide. Hydrogen peroxide is sometimes used as a preservative in milk designated for the manufacture of cheese. Catalase is added to the milk to neutralize the hydrogen peroxide just before the cheese-making process begins.

catalyst A substance that changes the rate of a chemical reaction without undergoing a change in itself. Catalysts may either increase or retard a reaction, but are generally added to speed it up. They are specific for particular processes. Enzymes function as catalysts, but in certain types of food processing, such as the conversion of vegetable oils to margarines by hydrogenation, metallic nickel or nickel-aluminum combinations may be also used.

celiac-sprue A chronic intestinal disorder characterized by diarrhea, steatorrhea, and malabsorption, leading to multiple nutritional deficiencies and arrest of growth in children. It is caused by an intolerance to gluten, a protein in wheat, barley, oats, and rye, and in food products containing these grains.

Gluten irritates the intestinal lining, which interferes with the absorption of fats, fat-soluble nutrients, and carbohydrates. Treatment includes a gluten-free diet with vitamin and mineral supplementation to correct the malnutrition and anemia. Cereal gluten is used in a myriad of commercial foods, ranging from canned soups and sauces to ice creams and processed meat products. Therefore, the gluten-sensitive person should read packaged food labels carefully to avoid adverse effects. See *malabsorption; malabsorption syndrome*.

cell The smallest structural and functional unit of an organism. A typical cell consists of a membrane enclosing a mass of protoplasm and a nucleus that controls reproduction and certain other functions. Cells vary considerably in size; a giant cell is about 1/1,000 of 1 in. in diameter, which is about 50 times as large as a bacterial cell. However, a single bacterium, so small that 200 would make a stack as thick as a sheet of paper, could contain 500 million molecules of proteins, fats, carbohydrates, and minerals, dissolved in 40 billion molecules of water.

cellulitis An acute inflammation of the deep tissues of the skin caused by a bacterial infection. The area of inflammation is tender, warm and sometimes has a dusky red to purple coloration.

cellulose A type of carbohydrate similar to starch in composition but with the sugar units organized in such a way that it cannot be digested by humans. The tough, fibrous cellulose molecules serve as a kind of skeleton for plants, providing strength and shape for their structures. Domestic animals like horses and cattle possess an enzyme that breaks down the cellulose molecule into glucose units; a cotton cellulose molecule is composed of a chain of as many as 9,000 glucose molecules. Although humans cannot digest cellulose, plant materials containing cellulose are beneficial to humans as they are the source of bulk, roughage, or fiber in the diet.

Celsius A temperature scale that is the equivalent of the old centigrade system, with the zero mark, or 0° Celsius, at the freezing point of water and 100° Celsius at the boiling point of water. It is used by scientists throughout the world and by the general population in countries that follow the metric system of measurement. The temperature scale is named for Anders Celsius, an eighteenth-century Swedish astronomer who introduced the centigrade temperature scale. Abbreviated °C.

cereal A term applied to the seeds of plants of the grass family, but generally limited to foods prepared from certain common cereal grains, such as barley, corn, oats, rice, wheat, millet, or rye. Cereals are sometimes called *farinaceous grains*, which simply means that they are rich in starch. See *enriched cereal products; refined cereal; whole-grain cereal*.

ceroid A yellow-to-brown insoluble fatty pigment found in the liver, nervous system, and muscles. It results from the fusion of unsaturated fatty acid residues and is found in both normal and diseased tissue.

cevitamic acid An alternative name for vitamin C, or ascorbic acid. The word *cevitamic* is an acronym derived from the combination of C, pronounced "cee," and vitamin.

chalaza The thick albuminous substance in an egg that extends from the yolk to the shell membrane and often appears as a white spiral.

cheilosis A skin disorder symptomatic of a riboflavin deficiency. It is characterized by the fissuring and dry scaling of the lips and angles of the mouth. Cheilosis may also accompany clinical signs of other B-vitamin deficiencies, such as lack of pyridoxine. Doctors usually treat the disorder with doses of B-complex vitamins.

chelation The process of forming a chemical compound or complex with a metallic ion. Chelation is used therapeutically to remove toxic metals from the body by causing them to form insoluble substances which cannot be absorbed from the intestine and therefore are excreted. Chelation may also occur naturally in the digestive tract, as when iron in the diet becomes bound to an insoluble complex and cannot be absorbed when needed by the body.

chemical score A method of rating the protein in a food. The content of each essential amino acid in a selected food is compared with the content of the same amino acid in the same quantity of a protein chosen as the standard, usually egg protein. The amino acid with the lowest percentage is the *limiting amino acid*, and this deficit is the chemical score. Also called *protein score*. See *limiting amino acid*.

chilblains A type of skin inflammation caused by exposure to cold temperatures. The feet, hands, ears, and nose are most commonly affected. Symptoms include a burning and itching sensation; the skin becomes mottled, swollen, and dark red. A contributing cause, in addition to the cold, is poor blood circulation in the affected areas. Although little can be done to improve circulation in the ears and nose, the hands and feet can be protected by exercise and the use of warm clothing in cold weather.

Chinese restaurant syndrome A temporary condition of discomfort caused by the ingestion of food containing monosodium glutamate (MSG). Symptoms include lightheadedness, a throbbing and sometimes aching head, backache, and a feeling of tightness or pressure about the jaws, neck, and shoulders. The sensitivity to MSG varies with different individuals. The disorder gets its name from the fact that food served in Chinese restaurants is often flavored liberally with MSG. The condition is not considered an allergic reaction, but a direct pharmacological effect. See *monosodium glutamate*.

chloride A form of the element chlorine that occurs in nature as an ion, or a negatively charged electrolyte, and is sometimes classified as a mineral. Chloride constitutes approximately 66 percent of the negatively charged ions in the extracellular fluids of humans. It is found in red blood cells and helps the body maintain its fluid and electrolyte balance and also plays a role in the adjustment of the acid-base balance of body fluids. An excess or deficiency of chloride can result in acidosis or alkalosis. In the digestive system, chloride forms a part of the hydrochloric acid of gastric juice. Table salt and meats are prime sources of chloride and humans rarely have a chloride-deficient diet.

chlorination A water treatment that disinfects and makes it safe for human consumption. Most organic matter and disease-causing bacteria are destroyed by the addition of chlorine to water supplies in amounts considered harmless for human consumption.

chlorine An element that occurs as a gas in nature but enters the body as part of a salt and functions in the tissues as an ion. Chlorine also plays an important role in the body's physiology as a component of hydrochloric acid in the gastric juice of the stomach. As an ion, it is one of the major ions of the body's extracellular fluid. Chlorine also helps maintain the acid-base balance of the blood, enters into the action of amylase enzymes, and assists in the absorption of iron and vitamin B-12 from the digestive tract.

cholecalciferol A natural form of vitamin D obtained from animal sources, such as egg yolk and butter, and from fish oils. It can also be produced synthetically. Also called *vitamin D-3*. See *vitamin D*.

cholesterol A pearly, fatlike substance found in animal fats and oils of foods consumed. It also occurs naturally in bile, blood, and tissues of the central nervous system and other organs. Cholesterol that enters the body through food is called *exogenous* cholesterol; that which the body synthesizes is *endogenous* cholesterol. Cholesterol accumulations in the arteries are responsible in part for the circulatory disease called *atherosclerosis*; cholesterol is also involved in the formation of gallstones.

On the positive side, cholesterol is an essential component of cell membranes and is a precursor of vitamin D and certain steroid hormones, particularly the sex hormones. Cholesterol is technically an alcohol, despite its association with fatty foods. The major dietary sources of cholesterol include eggs, liver, sweetbreads, oysters, butter, and cheddar cheese, followed by meats, fish, and poultry. Vegetable products, such as margarines made from corn oil or other vegetable oils, do not contain cholesterol because the substance simply does not occur in plants. Because the body produces its own cholesterol, it is not possible to have a cholesterol-free life. However, doctors usually advise people who are likely candidates for cardiovascular disorders to avoid the exogenous, or dietary, types of cholesterol.

cholic acid One of several bile acids. It is formed in the liver from cholesterol and plays an important role in the digestive processes. Cholic acid also becomes a part of one of the bile salts that help break up large droplets of fat into smaller droplets.

choline A vitamin that is a member of the B-complex. It exists in many kinds of plant and animal tissues and is also produced synthetically. Choline is a basic component of lecithin and other phospholipids important for normal body functions. In addition, it helps prevent the accumulation of fats in the liver when diets are rich in fats and carbohydrates but deficient in proteins. Choline aids in the metabolism of fats as a constituent of bile, where it was first discovered in the early nineteenth century. It also plays a vital role in nerve functions as a precursor of acetylcholine, a substance that helps nerve impulses travel through the body.

The choline molecule contains three units called *methyl groups*, each composed of one carbon and three hydrogen atoms, which are split off by the body's chemical factories and used in the formation of several substances synthesized by the body. These are the hormone epinephrine (or adrenaline), the energy-rich compound called creatine that is needed for muscle metabolism and certain waste products that require methyl groups before being excreted in the urine. The body synthesizes some choline, but usually less than the amount required by humans. Therefore, many nutrition experts recommend that foods containing choline, such as egg yolks, be included in the diet. Other sources are beef liver, peas, beans, soybeans, and milk. Some vegetables contain choline but fruits are not an adequate source.

chromium A mineral that is a required nutrient for normal human health. Its physiological role is associated with glucose metabolism and it is believed to be needed to improve the effectiveness of insulin in making glucose available to body tissue cells. Some studies indicate chromium is also involved in the metabolism of proteins and fats. A deficiency of chromium is linked to retarded development in young people. Because levels of the element decline with age it is believed to be a factor in longevity. Good sources include meat, milk, poultry, fish, and shellfish, particularly raw oysters. Also called *glucose tolerance factor*.

cirrhosis of the liver An inflammation of the liver marked by degeneration of the liver cells, which are replaced by fibrous and nodular tissue. The disease is associated with metabolic disorders and disturbances in fluid and electrolyte balance. Early signs and symptoms include loss of appetite, weight loss, fatigue, and lowered resistance to infection. If the disease is not controlled, later signs include a red coloration of the palms of the hands, spider-shaped blood vessel markings of the skin, loss of body hair, and testicular atrophy. Treatment involves restriction of alcoholic beverages, a high-protein, high-carbohydrate diet, and vitamin supplements.

citric acid   One of the most common acids present in fruits and vegetables. Small amounts of citric acid are found, even in foods that are considered base, or alkaline. Citric acid content ranges from about 1/100 of 1 percent in celery and cucumbers to about 4 percent in lemons. Oranges and grapefruit contain approximately 1 percent citric acid, but currants, blueberries, cranberries, and red raspberries often contain higher amounts. It is a relatively mild acid used as a flavoring and buffer in soft drinks, bakery products, and medicines. Citric acid can be manufactured synthetically from sugar; it is produced during the digestion of food as a stage in metabolism. Citric acid can be completely metabolized to carbon dioxide and water.

citric acid cycle   See *Krebs cycle*.

citrulline   One of the nonessential amino acids. It is involved in the production of urea.

clarifying agents   Compounds used in the production of some beverages and vinegar to remove minute particles and traces of copper or iron. These substances include tannin, gelatin, and albumin.

clear liquid diet   A diet that consists of clear soups and broths, tea, coffee, gelatin preparations, and water. It is mainly used to sustain patients who have just undergone certain types of surgery. The patient may also be given apple juice, grape juice, or a carbonated beverage, such as ginger ale, if the attending physician approves.

club soda   See *soda water*.

coal tar   A thick, black liquid produced by the distillation of coal, sometimes as a by-product in the manufacture of coke and coal gas. Specific chemicals that can be isolated from coal tar have been used in the production of certain food additives and medications.

cobalamin   See *vitamin B-12*.

cobalt   A mineral required in small amounts because it is a component of vitamin B-12, which in turn is needed for the formation of red blood cells. A deficit of vitamin B-12 can result in pernicious anemia, but cobalt cannot be used to correct the condition. Cobalt absorption from the digestive tract is associated with the level of iron absorption, which suggests a related physiological mechanism. An excess of cobalt in the diet can result in thyroid disorders and congestive heart failure. The body needs only about 3 parts per 10-million of cobalt, so a deficiency is very unlikely in a normal human body.

cobblestone tongue The common name for a disorder of the tongue in which the papillae, or tiny nipple-shaped projections, become red and swollen. The cause is usually a vitamin B-complex deficiency.

cod-liver oil An oil obtained from the livers of codfish and one of the best sources of fish oils. It is rich in vitamins A and D and is used as a source of those vitamins in some vitamin supplements.

coenzyme A substance that functions with another substance as a catalyst for a chemical reaction in the body tissues. Vitamins, particularly vitamins in the B-complex group, are coenzymes that unite with a large protein molecule, called an *apoenzyme*. Apoenzymes produce a specific reaction, such as a step in the metabolism of a food element or conversion of a food element residue into a compound that can be easily excreted through the kidneys. The combination of a coenzyme and an apoenzyme is sometimes called a holoenzyme. An example of a vitamin coenzyme is pantothenic acid, which is sometimes identified as coenzyme A.

coenzyme A See *pantothenic acid.*

cofactor A substance or process that requires one or more additional factors in order to function properly. An example of a cofactor is a coenzyme.

coffee A beverage made from the roasted seeds of the fruit of one of the varieties of coffee trees that grow in the mountainous terrain of tropical countries. When ripe, the fruit of the coffee tree is a bright red cherry color. When the pulp of the fruit is removed, two oval-shaped seeds, flat on one side, remain and are called *coffee beans*. The main pharmacologically active ingredient of coffee is the central nervous system stimulant, *caffeine*. Coffee beans contain small amounts of B vitamins and some minerals but their thiamine content is destroyed in the roasting process.

coffee whiteners Nondairy creamers used in place of a dairy product for adding to coffee and other beverages. They contain mixtures of vegetable fat, protein, sugar, stabilizers, flavor, and color. See *dairy food substitutes.*

cold sore A sore or blister caused by the infection of a common virus called *Herpes simplex*. The sore is actually a cluster of tiny blisters or swellings on the lip or another area of skin or mucous membrane. The watery blisters are painful but usually erupt after a few days, to be replaced by a crust. The virus is usually a permanent resident of the body and makes its appearance during a period of physical or emotional stress, such as overexposure to sunlight, an allergic reaction, or anxiety. Also called *fever blister*.

colitis An inflammation of the colon, the lower end of the large intestine. One of the more common forms of colitis is *spastic colitis* or *irritable bowel syndrome*, which is marked by cramplike pains and constipation that alternates with and is gradually dominated by diarrhea. Causes include emotional distress and anxiety, but improper eating habits are also a major factor. Treatment often includes relatively bland meals served without strong seasonings, caffeine beverages, or alcohol, and eaten in an attractive, serene, pleasant setting. Proper exercise, avoidance of emotional conflicts, and the use of sedatives or other medications may also be a part of the treatment.

collagen An albuminous type of protein that serves as a supportive tissue in skin, tendons, cartilage, bone, and connective tissues in general. It appears in animal tissues as white fibers that are flexible but inelastic and become gelatinous when boiled in water.

colostrum The first milk secreted by the mother's breasts following the delivery of her child. Colostrum is richer in lactoprotein and lactoalbumin than the regular breast milk produced later. Colostrum also has a laxative effect on the child that helps move the meconium, a mass of material that accumulates in the fetal intestine during gestation, from the digestive tract.

common cold A relatively mild but acute and highly contagious upper respiratory tract infection transmitted by a virus. Symptoms include sneezing, cough, nasal discharge, watering eyes, and sometimes a fever, usually lasting from 1 to 2 weeks. At least 20 different viruses are known to produce common cold symptoms in humans, usually when they are in a state of lowered resistance. Having a cold does not make one immune to future infections and there is no preventive vaccine. The recommended therapy is to take a common cold seriously and try to avoid complications by going to bed, keeping warm, drinking plenty of fluids, and avoiding contact with other people.

complementary proteins A term applied to combinations of proteins that together contribute the essential amino acids, although none of the individual protein sources provides all of them. Examples are found in the diets of people in Third World countries who cannot afford the best sources of proteins, such as eggs, milk, and meat. A meal of complementary proteins might include beans and corn. Beans contribute the essential amino acids missing from corn, and corn provides the essential amino acids not found in beans.

complete protein A protein food source that contains all the essential amino acids. Eggs and milk are examples of complete proteins. Complete protein quality can be altered by food preparation methods that interfere with digestibility and thus the ability of the body to absorb the essential nutrients of the complete protein.

compound A substance composed of two or more materials or chemical elements. The elements entering into a chemical compound generally become altered in the union so that their individual original characteristics are replaced by those of the compound. Table salt, or sodium chloride, for example, is a simple compound of sodium, a highly reactive metal, and chlorine, a poisonous gas; water is a compound of two kinds of gas, hydrogen and oxygen.

congener A term meaning something that resembles another in content or that produces similar effects. It is also a name that is sometimes applied to flavoring additives used in alcoholic beverages. Many people are sensitive to the congeners used to flavor bourbon, rum, and other types of liquor and they feel the effects later as a "hangover."

connective tissue A type of fibrous body tissue that consists mainly of long fibers embedded in substances outside cell membranes. The fibers are composed of collagen and other chemicals that determine the texture of the tissue, which in some cases may be soft and rubbery or hard and rigid. Scar tissue is an example of common connective tissue. Other examples are found in bones, tissues like tendons that attach muscles to bones, the walls of blood vessels, and structures that support and connect internal organs.

consistency modification A change made in the kind and amount of fiber or cellulose content of a diet, or in a residue-containing food.

constipation A condition in which fecal matter is not soft enough to move easily through the bowel or moves so infrequently as to cause discomfort. In the absence of a disorder, such as a hernia or tumor obstructing the bowel, or a hormonal disorder like hypothyroidism, the movement of food wastes through the bowel is primarily a matter of personal eating and life style habits and individual constitutional variations. Custom is also a factor, according to studies that show the "transit time" for food wastes to move through the bowel is much slower in European populations than in African or Asian countries where the usual diet contains more bulk. Emotional tension can also be a cause of constipation.

consumer product labeling A program instituted by the U.S. government requiring processed and packaged foods to carry labels showing the nutrient values of food items. The information on a food label shows the nutrient values of the food in terms of the U.S. Recommended Daily Allowances (RDAs); the exact information depends on the food item, whether it is enriched or fortified, and whether any particular claims are made by the manufacturer regarding the nutritional quality of the food. Some information may be added voluntarily by the manufacturer, such as optional vitamins and minerals. Sodium or cholesterol content may be included on some labels. The manufacturer is expected to be able to prove any nutritional claims on a label.

consumption units Quantities used to express the amount and kind of food or of nutrients present in foods consumed per person, group, or on some other selected basis.

contact dermatitis A skin inflammation that results from contact with an irritating substance, such as a chemical used in clothing manufacture or a toxic plant material like poison ivy. Numerous substances in the environment, from hair sprays and deodorants to evergreen trees and onions, can produce contact dermatitis in a person who is sensitive to the chemicals or substances in them.

controlled study A scientific experiment in which as many factors as possible are controlled to reduce the risk of error in the study results. Generally, in a study with laboratory animals, each experimental animal is matched as to sex, age, weight, heredity, and other aspects, with a "control" animal. During the experiment, both the experimental and control animals will eat the same food, live in the same area, and lead essentially the same kind of life, with the exception that the experimental animals will receive one food or drug item not given to the controls. When the study is completed, any effects found in the experimental animals can be attributed to the item tested.

convenience foods Semiprepared or ready-to-eat foods in which one or more steps in preparation have been completed before the product is offered for sale. See *junk food*.

cooking oils Vegetable oils processed specifically for cooking or frying, such as oils sold to hotels and restaurants for deep-fat frying. Cooking oils are generally alkali-refined, bleached, deodorized, and in some cases, "winterized" so they will not crystallize when refrigerated. One exception is virgin olive oil, which is not deodorized because it is expected to have an aroma. Bleaching to give the oil a lighter color may vary in degree according to the market, since consumers in some areas prefer a cooking oil that is not lighter than olive oil in color. Cooking oils are usually labeled as such to distinguish them from salad oils.

copper A mineral required by the human body in small amounts for a variety of functions, including its role in the production of the skin pigment called *melanin*.

Copper is either a cofactor or otherwise associated with several enzymes. It is required for the absorption of iron and its incorporation into the hemoglobin molecules of red blood cells. Copper is needed for the formation of a substance called *elastin*, which is a protein with elastic qualities used by the body in connective tissue. It also participates in the formation of myelin, a fatty protective sheath that covers many of the important nerve fibers. All of these jobs are done with as little as 100 mg. of copper, which is approximately 1/300 of 1 oz.

The body normally loses between 2 and 5 percent of its copper supply each day, an amount that must be replaced by a diet that contains up to 15 to 20 mg. of the element because only a minor fraction of the total intake is absorbed. The liver of a newborn infant contains between 5 and 10 times the amount of copper present in the liver of an older human, suggesting that nature is aware that milk is not a good food source of copper and the child needs extra reserves of the substance to carry it through the nursing period of its life. Many cases of copper deficiency have been found among infants whose diet consisted almost entirely of cow's milk well past the weaning stage.

Getting the right amount of copper in the diet is very important. Too much copper can lead to personality changes, including psychotic behavior. Too little copper can also alter behavior patterns as well as cause a form of anemia. Fruits, vegetables, eggs, cereals, seafood, and liver are good food sources of copper.

corrinoids The name of substances that are chemical cousins of cyanocobalamin, or vitamin B-12. However, corrinoids are not equal in potency to vitamin B-12.

cortisone A hormone produced by the adrenal glands and which can also be manufactured from plant substances. Natural cortisone is converted by the body to a slightly different substance, *hydrocortisone* or *cortisol*, in order to increase its effectiveness in the body. Cortisone is administered therapeutically in the treatment of certain disorders, such as rheumatoid arthritis.

cross-linking A process by which protein molecules in the skin and other organs become linked in structural meshes that reduce the flexibility of the tissue. The toughness of skin in older people is a result of protein cross-linking.

crystals Solid objects that have naturally flat surfaces. Table salt is an example of a crystal. Large crystals are usually composed of smaller units of the same substance, arranged systematically and evenly spaced along a theoretical lattice pattern. Many substances that appear as dissolved materials in a fluid become crystal deposits when the temperature is reduced or the amount of solvent falls below the level needed to keep the salt in solution. Many food products, such as vegetable oils, contain substances that prevent the formation of crystals.

cyanide A usually toxic chemical found in small quantities in the human body as a result of the metabolism of foods containing cyanogens, such as apricots, cherries, plums, sweet potatoes, lima beans, and peas. Oil of bitter almonds also contains cyanide. A lethal dose is approximately 30 mg. for an adult human, but death has occurred in children from chewing as few as five apricot pits.

cyanocobalamin See *vitamin B-12*.

cyanogens Substances present in some foods that produce biologically significant quantities of cyanide. Called *cyanogenetic glycosides*, they are found in some fruit seeds, including apricot kernels, some species of beans, and a variety of other plants. When the raw plant material is eaten, enzymes release the poison. Cooking does not always prevent this release. See *cyanide*.

cyclamates A group of artificial sweeteners banned in the United States and certain other countries as a result of studies conducted in the 1960s which reportedly showed that laboratory rats fed cyclamates developed bladder tumors. See *Delaney Clause*.

cyclic AMP (cyclic adenosine monophosphate) A vital substance produced by the action of the enzyme adenyl cyclase in cell membranes on adenosine triphosphate (ATP) in the cytoplasm of cells. Cyclic AMP controls the functions of DNA molecules in various life functions and interacts with vitamins and other nutrients and human metabolites. It also serves as a "messenger" that assists many hormones in delivering their activating signal to their target organs.

cystathionine A substance produced during the conversion of the amino acid methionine to cysteine. It is an important component of many protein molecules. An inherited metabolic disorder is marked by a deficiency of an enzyme needed to complete the process; cystathione accumulates in the body, resulting in mental retardation, abnormal bone growth, acidosis, and other health problems.

cysteine A nonessential amino acid that is utilized by the body in its production of insulin molecules and the keratin cells of hair structure. Like cystine, it can be formed by the body from the essential amino acid methionine.

cystine One of the nonessential amino acids. It can be manufactured in the body from the essential amino acid methionine. Cystine is also the primary sulfur-containing component of protein molecules. In a disorder called *Fanconi's disease*, one of the symptoms is an accumulation of cystine in tissues throughout the body.

cytochromes A group of proteins that contain iron and are widely distributed in plant and animal tissues. They aid in the respiration of individual cells within the various organ tissues.

d

daily food guide The name of a system developed by the U.S. Department of Agriculture to help people with a minimum amount of knowledge about nutrition plan balanced meals by including items from each of the basic four food groups.

dairy food substitutes A group of foods that includes imitation cream or coffee whiteners, imitation cheese, and ice cream. These substitutes may contain milk components even though they are called *nondairy products*. They may also differ markedly in composition from the product they resemble.

DDT A chemical shorthand name for *dichlorodiphenyltrichloroethane*, a highly toxic insecticide that affects the central nervous system, causing tremors, extreme excitability, muscular weakness, and convulsions. A dose of more than ⅔ of 1 oz. can be fatal. DDT has been banned in the United States for nearly 10 years because it enters the food chain and can accumulate in fatty tissues of humans and foods eaten by humans. Also, because DDT has a half-life of 15 years, one-half the DDT used anywhere in the world in 1972 will still be in the environment in 1987 and one-fourth will still be around in the year 2002.

deaminization The process of removing the amino unit from an amino acid molecule. The term is also used to describe the splitting-off of an amino unit, a combination of one nitrogen and two hydrogen atoms, from any molecule. Deaminization is a common occurrence in the human body while amino acids in the diet are being metabolized. The process may be one step in building nonessential amino acids from parts of essential amino acids, or simply a routine procedure for disposing of leftover amino acids by breaking them down into bits of fuel to be burned for their energy content. The nitrogen portion cannot be burned and must be converted to urea to be excreted. Also called *deamination*.

decarboxylation A process in the metabolism of amino acids in which a carbon dioxide unit is split away from the amino acid molecule. Decarboxylation is often a step in the creation of a new substance, as when the amino acid histidine is converted to histamine. Pyridoxine and thiamine participate as coenzymes in certain decarboxylation activities.

deficiency diseases Disorders or disease conditions with characteristic clinical signs caused by a lack of specific nutrients, and which can be cured by supplying the missing substances, such as fatty acids, trace elements, or vitamins. Examples include *beriberi, iron-deficiency anemia,* and *scurvy.* See these entries; see also *subclinical deficiency.*

deglutition A medical term for the act of swallowing. The process is partly voluntary and partly involuntary. The voluntary aspect involves using the tongue and cheek muscles to move the chewed food to the back of the mouth. The involuntary action is the movement of the epiglottis over the trachea, or windpipe, to prevent food from entering that opening: instead, it directs the food into the top of the esophagus, which leads to the stomach.

degradation The process in body chemistry in which a complex molecule is reduced to a simpler substance by splitting off one or more groups of atoms. See *deaminization; decarboxylation.*

dehydration The loss of or removal of water from the body, a part of the body, or a food item. The normal loss of water from the body through urination, the digestive tract, the lungs, and skin totals more than 2 qt., or 2 liters, daily; it is normally replaced by an equivalent amount of fluids, such as water, beverages, and foods containing moisture. Body dehydration can occur through fever, diarrhea, acidosis, injuries such as burns, surgery, and various diseases that cause a loss of abnormal amounts of fluids. Dehydration of foods is a common practice in packaging and preserving processes, as in the manufacture of instant coffees.

dehydroascorbic acid A form of ascorbic acid, or vitamin C, caused by oxidation of ascorbic acid. Although dehydroascorbic acid still has antiscurvy qualities, it is fairly unstable and can easily undergo a loss of its vitamin potency by exposure to copper or iron, heat, an alkaline medium, or air and sunlight. Orange juice that has undergone extensive processing may have suffered such a loss of vitamin quality.

dehydroretinol The chemical name for vitamin A-2. See *vitamin A.*

Delaney Clause A clause added to the 1958 Food Additives Amendment to the Federal Food, Drug and Cosmetic Act. It requires the U.S. Food and Drug

Administration to ban any food or food additive that has been shown to produce cancer in laboratory animals by any "appropriate test." The legislation has been the source of controversy because of the difficulty of translating results of laboratory tests with animals into terms of normal human food consumption or determining whether any laboratory test is otherwise appropriate. Also called *Cancer Clause.*

delirium tremens A severe form of alcohol withdrawal syndrome, marked by attacks of anxiety, confusion, inability to sleep, profuse sweating, and profound depression. The pulse rate increases to more than 100 per minute and the temperature rises to at least 100°. In severe cases, pulse rate and temperature may go even higher. Hallucinations and illusions, often involving animals, are experienced, particularly in dim light. Typical of the confusion and disorientation of the delirium tremens patient is the mistaken belief that he is at his job, even though he may be in a hospital, so that he becomes engaged in some activity that he believes is job related.

demineralization The loss of calcium from the bones during periods of calcium deficiency diets. The parathyroid hormone system regulates the amount of calcium in the bloodstream, where it is made available to the neuromuscular and other body systems. When the calcium level in the blood falls below a certain level, the mineral is "shaved" from the body's skeleton. When there is an excess of calcium in the body, however, the parathyroid hormone arranges for it to be excreted through the urinary tract, the digestive tract, or in perspiration through the skin.

demulcent Any soothing, bland substance given a poisoning victim in addition to fluids administered to dilute or neutralize the poison. Demulcents, such as milk, egg white, or olive oil, coat the lining of the digestive tract so the poison is less likely to be absorbed into the blood.

dental plaque A film of bacteria and other substances that accumulates on the surface of the teeth. Plaque may include food debris and the waste products of bacterial metabolism.

dental ulcer An ulcer that develops along the sides or under the tongue, where the tongue rubs against a protruding tooth or poorly fitted dentures. The dental ulcer usually has a distinct appearance of a trough or groove, showing the path of friction, rather than the rounded area usually associated with an ulcer. If treated early, the ulcer ordinarily heals by itself within a few weeks. Untreated dental ulcers can develop into cancers.

deoxycholic acid One of the bile acids. It forms soluble complexes with fatty acids as a step toward enabling them to be absorbed from the small intestine.

Deoxycholic acid also combines with another substance in the digestive tract to form one of the bile salts.

deoxyribonucleic acid A complex molecule that consists of two spiral chains of molecules of four basic substances—adenine, cytosine, guanine, and thymine—plus phosphoric acid and a sugar called *deoxyribose*. These molecules contain the genetic information for the reproduction of the species and are found in the body cells of all living organisms, including most viruses, some of which consist of little more than deoxyribonucleic acid molecules. They also contain the pattern or instructions for the formation of proteins, enzymes, and other structural and functional units of life. Abbreviated *DNA*.

dermatitis Any inflammation of the skin. Causes may be excessive heat or cold; infectious agents; contact with an irritant, for example, poison ivy or an acid; sunlight; or a systemic disorder such as eczema. Certain drugs can also be a cause of dermatitis. Hives is a form of dermatitis associated with an allergic reaction or hypersensitivity to a substance that may be present in a food item.

dermis The layer of skin immediately below the epidermis. The dermis generally is much thicker than the epidermis and contains connective tissue, nerves, blood vessels, and ducts for oil and sweat glands. Beneath the dermis is a third skin layer, the subcutaneous tissue containing numerous fat cells, and, in some skin areas such as the scalp, the hair roots. See *epidermis*.

desalination Partial or complete removal of salts from seawater or brackish water so that it can be used for household or agricultural purposes. A number of methods for purification are used, including distillation and solar evaporation.

dextran A large sugar molecule produced by the action of a strain of bacteria on sucrose. Dextran is used therapeutically to extend the blood plasma of a patient, and in food manufacture as a stabilizer for syrups, ice creams, and candies.

dextrin One of the by-products of the action of certain body enzymes on starch. For example, an enzyme in saliva, *ptyalin*, splits starch molecules into dextrin and maltose while the starchy food is being chewed. Another enzyme in the pancreas performs a similar function on starches that reach the small intestine without already being broken into smaller units. Dextrins can also be manufactured from starch by artificial processes that use heat or acids, or both. Wheat dextrin, for example, is produced by the baking of bread and contributes to the formation of crust on a bread loaf.

dextrose A form of glucose. The term is composed from parts of the words *dextrorotatory*, which refers to the direction in which the dextrose molecule turns rays of light, and *glucose*. About 80 percent of all simple sugar in food, particularly fruit sugars, is dextrose. It is less sweet than table sugar, or sucrose. Dextrose is used as an additive in soft drinks, to give them body, and other processed foods.

DHHS An abbreviation for the U.S. Department of Health and Human Services, which formerly was the Department of Health, Education, and Welfare.

diabetes mellitus A metabolic disorder in which the body is unable to make effective use of carbohydrate foods in the diet because of a defect in the insulin mechanism.

The inability to metabolize carbohydrates is normally complicated by disorders of protein and fat metabolism; the defect in carbohydrate metabolism results in an accelerated consumption of fat for fuel so that fat by-products accumulate in the blood, producing symptoms of acidosis, ketosis, and coma.

There is no single cause for diabetes mellitus and the disruption of the body's insulin mechanism. Among possible causes are an insufficient production of insulin from the cells of the pancreas, an excessive demand for insulin by the body tissues, and a loss of insulin effectiveness because of such factors as the presence of insulin antagonists that interfere with the function of the hormone. The disease tends to occur more often in women, in people who have a family history of diabetes, in people over age 40, those with a type of obesity in which abnormal fat deposits are located above the waistline, and in persons who have experienced a viral infection that affected the pancreas.

In the absence of enough insulin to enable the body tissues to use the sugar entering the body, the diabetic patient suffers from a form of malnutrition, regardless of how much food he eats. He experiences weakness and fatigue and the unused sugar in his blood is excreted in the urine. The kidneys, heart, and blood vessels may be damaged and the nervous system affected, with a gradual loss of vision. Diabetes is controlled by diet, exercise to regulate the amount of body fuel, and the administration of insulin. See *food exchanges; insulin; diabetic diet.*

diabetic diet A diet for diabetes mellitus patients that emphasizes maximum intake of essential nutrients with a minimum of concentrated sweets. The precise diabetic diet is usually ordered by the patient's physician. Although the diet is somewhat flexible because of the use of food exchange lists, meals are consumed at prescribed times, particularly when insulin injections are administered. There are six basic exchange lists for diabetics, one each for milk, vegetables, fruits, breads, meats, and fats. Each item on an exchange list is measured in terms of protein, fat, carbohydrate, and calories.

dialysis A method of removing from the blood by artificial means the substances normally excreted in the urine. It is used mainly when a person has suffered kidney failure. The process involves the use of a semipermeable membrane similar to the surrounding body tissue cells that permits certain small molecules, such as glucose and urea, to pass through tiny openings while preventing the movement of large molecules, like proteins.

One kind of dialyzer, called the *hemodialyzer*, or *artificial kidney*, uses a membrane made of a synthetic material, such as cellophane. Blood is removed from an artery in the arm of the patient and routed through tubing to the dialyzing machine which indirectly "washes" the blood on one side of the membrane while a dialyzing solution on the other side collects the waste materials that filter through it. The clean blood is then recirculated back into the patient's body.

A second kind of dialysis equipment uses the peritoneal cavity of the patient, which is a space between two natural membranes that separate the abdominal organs from the abdominal wall. The peritoneal membrane serves as the filtering device and the dialyzing solution is pumped into the cavity, then pumped out again when the blood has been cleaned. In addition to the use of dialysis for persons with impaired kidney function, the technique can be used to remove certain poisonous substances from the bloodstream.

diaphragmatic hernia See *hiatus hernia*.

diarrhea The abnormally rapid movement of fecal material through the intestine, caused by irritation of the bowel lining by an infectious agent or toxic substance, an emotional disorder, or related causes. Symptoms include frequent watery stools, possibly streaked with blood; weakness; and abdominal cramps. Because diarrhea results in loss of fluid and nutrients, prolonged or repeated attacks of this disorder can be marked by dehydration, malnutrition, and anemia.

diastase An enzyme complex produced by the germination of grain seeds, particularly barley, that is capable of converting starch into sugar. Diastase is involved in the malting process important in brewing, baking, and other types of food manufacture.

diastolic The minimum blood pressure measured with a sphygmomanometer, the instrument commonly used by medical personnel to measure blood pressure. Diastolic pressure, which is written as the lower of the two numbers that record one's blood pressure, represents the pressure when the heart is resting between contractions. See *blood pressure; systolic*.

dibasic ammonium phosphate An odorless white powder used in baking, brewing, sugar processing, and certain special foods that are made slightly acidic by its presence.

dicoumarin The name of an anticoagulant drug that acts by blocking four steps of the blood-clotting process. It is an antivitamin to vitamin K. Dicoumarin was discovered during research in the 1920s to determine the cause of a fatal bleeding disease that affected cattle after they ate sweet clover; the cause was found to be dicoumarin produced by the clover. Also called *dicumarol*.

diet The combinations of foods and beverages consumed by a person during a given period, particularly combinations designed to include or exclude certain nutrients or amounts of nutrients. A diet may be planned on a day-to-day basis, for a specified period of time, or as a continuing health regimen. An elimination diet planned to detect a food allergy may be continued until the allergen has been identified. See the entries for descriptions of specific diets.

dietary history A detailed account of the kind, estimated amount, and preparation methods of the usual daily food intake for an individual, obtained in interview by a health professional, most commonly a dietitian. A sufficient period of time, more than 24 hr. must be covered to obtain an accurate record.

dietetic beverages A term applied to soft drinks in which an artificial sweetener is used as a substitute for sugar or corn syrup. Regular soft drinks generally contain between 8 and 14 percent sugar. Cyclamates were commonly used as a nonnutritive sweetener in soft drinks in the United States until 1969, when saccharin was authorized by the U.S. Food and Drug Administration as a replacement for cyclamates, which had been found to be a cause of cancer in laboratory animals. Aspartame was introduced as an artificial sweetener for soft drinks in 1984. When an artificial sweetener is used in a dietetic beverage, an additional additive, such as carboxymethyl cellulose or pectin, may be used to give the drink the body that would normally be provided by the use of a sugar syrup in the beverage. See *aspartame, Delaney Clause*.

dietetic foods Foods intended for use in special diets that have had their nutrient content modified in some way. Foods with a sugar substitute or without added sugar were the first to be marketed for diabetics. Now there are dietetic products for many special diets, such as low fat, gluten free, and for those who are allergic to specific substances.

diethylstilbestrol A synthetic sex hormone that has been used as a livestock feed additive to stimulate meat production at a lower cost per animal. The hormone increases the protein and water content of the meat while decreasing the proportion of muscle fat in beef. Because of evidence that diethylstilbestrol can cause cancer in humans and laboratory animals, livestock feeders are required to discontinue the use of the hormone in feed for at least 2 weeks before the animal is scheduled to be slaughtered.

dietitian A person who is professionally qualified to provide nutritional care. In the United States, the American Dietetic Association is responsible for qualifications and registration of dietitians.

digestibility A measure of the proportion of food eaten that can actually be absorbed and utilized by the body systems. The digestibility, or completeness of digestion, varies with different food elements and food sources. Of the protein in animal foods, for example, digestibility averages around 97 percent, compared to only 78 percent for dried legumes. Carbohydrate digestibility ranges from a high of 98 percent in animal foods down to 90 percent for fruits. The digestibility of fats is around 90 percent for all types of food sources except animal foods, in which case it is 95 percent.

digestion The process of converting chemical substances in food into chemical substances that can be utilized by the tissues of the body.
    The digestive process in humans takes place in the alimentary canal, or digestive system, a tube that extends from the mouth to the anus and is technically outside the body although completely surrounded by organs and tissues of other body systems. Digestion involves the physical breaking up of food materials by churning, diluting, dissolving, and splitting complex molecules of protein, fats, and carbohydrates into simple amino acid, fatty acid, and sugar units. The process is aided by enzymes and secretions from salivary glands, the liver, gall bladder, and pancreas. Vitamins participate in certain digestive functions as enzyme cofactors.
    Digestion begins in the mouth, where chewing breaks food into smaller pieces that are moistened and exposed to the enzyme ptyalin, which begins starch breakdown. In the stomach, the chewed food is exposed to hydrochloric acid and several digestive enzymes—rennin, pepsin, and lipase—as it is churned for a period ranging from 2 to 6 hr. From the stomach, the food, now whipped into a semifluid substance called *chyme*, is further exposed to the action of liver bile, steapsin, amylopsin, trypsin, chymotrypsin, and a peptidase from pancreatic juices, plus erepsin, maltase, sucrase, and lactase in intestinal digestive juices. By the time the meal reaches the large intestine, digestion and absorption of food is more than 90 percent complete. In the large intestine, most of the remaining water is absorbed and the food residue is formed into feces to be excreted. The forward movement of the digestive process after food enters the esophagus is caused by *peristalsis*, or contractions of digestive muscles.

digestive juices The various fluids secreted into the digestive tract between the mouth and the small intestine to aid in the breakdown of complex substances in food elements.
    The digestive juices include *ptyalin*, an enzyme in the saliva secreted into

the mouth by three pairs of salivary glands. Ptyalin begins the digestive process by breaking cooked starch into maltose molecules.

The stomach contains three enzymes plus hydrochloric acid in a fluid known as *gastric juice*. The enzymes are *rennin*, which coagulates the milk protein so it can be acted on by a second enzyme, *pepsin*, which breaks down protein molecules into smaller units. The third stomach enzyme, *lipase*, begins the digestion of fats into fatty acids and glycerol.

In the small intestine, the four enzymes found in intestinal juice include *erepsin*, which continues breaking proteins into amino acids, and three carbohydrate enzymes, *maltase, sucrase,* and *lactase*, which split maltose, sucrose, and lactose, respectively, into glucose and other simple sugar molecules. *Bile* from the bile duct enters the small intestine along with a group of enzymes from the pancreas through a shared conduit. The bile, produced in the liver, emulsifies fats while *steapsin* from the pancreas breaks the emulsified fat into fatty acids and glycerol. A carbohydrate enzyme from the pancreas, *amylopsin*, continues the metabolism of starches begun in the mouth. And three other substances from the pancreas—*trypsin, chymotrypsin,* and *carboxypolypeptidase* work on protein molecules, breaking them into amino acids or amino acid chains called *peptides*, which are finally split by erepsin. See *digestion; digestibility*.

digestive microbes Microscopic organisms that inhabit the digestive tract and aid in certain functions, such as vitamin activities. The synthesis of biotin, folic acid, niacin, thiamine, vitamin B-12, and vitamin K are believed to be dependent in whole or in part on the presence of digestive tract microbes. Evidence of the need for certain friendly bacteria in the digestive tract is found in the fact that nutritional deficiencies can result from elimination of the microbes by the use of antibiotic medications.

digitalis A heart tonic drug extracted from the leaf of the digitalis, or foxglove, plant. Digitalis is prescribed for congestive heart failure because it strengthens contractions of the heart muscle while slowing the rate; the more efficient heart function helps eliminate excess body fluid that otherwise would accumulate in the body. Digitalis is one of several folk remedies once grown in "witch gardens" and dispensed without a prescription before it was "discovered" by the medical profession.

diglycerides Fats composed of a glycerol molecule attached to two fatty acids. Diglycerides have emulsifying properties that put them in demand as additives for shortenings and other food products.

dioctyl sodium sulfosuccinate A long mouthful of words for a wetting agent used as a food additive. A wetting agent is a substance added to things that are hard to wet when used in food processing, for example, powders like fumaric acid added to soft drink preparations, or cocoa butter added to canned milk products. If these substances are not treated with a wetting agent, they will not disperse in the liquid. Abbreviated: *DSS*.

disaccharidase An enzyme that splits *disaccharides*, or two-unit sugars, into simple sugars like glucose. This enzyme is important because a deficiency of disaccharidase in the small intestine can be the cause of sugar malabsorption, marked by intestinal cramps, intestinal gas, and diarrhea. Lactase deficiency is an example of a disaccharidase defect that results in lactose intolerance, or the inability to digest milk sugar.

disaccharide Any of the sugar molecules formed by a combination of two simple sugars, such as glucose. One example of a disaccharide is sucrose.

discrimination A term used to express the ability of the body to make a selective choice between calcium and strontium in their absorption and retention. The two minerals are alike in some ways, including metabolism, and a tendency to occur together in foods and to accumulate in bones. It has been found that the body will discriminate against strontium, choosing calcium instead, and that as calcium intake increases, strontium absorption decreases. This is seen as a protective measure to prevent a large build-up of strontium.

disodium guanylate A flavor enhancer and a chemical cousin of monosodium glutamate (MSG). The two additives are often used together in processed vegetables, meats, and soups because they have a synergistic effect on each other, producing a greater effect in combination than when used alone. Abbreviated *GMP*.

disodium ionosinate A flavor enhancer that is related to and functions like *monosodium glutamate* (MSG) and *disodium guanylate* (GMP). See these entries. Abbreviated *IMP*.

disodium phosphate A food additive used in many products as an emulsifier, a buffer, and as a sequestrant to stabilize colors and odors. In the manufacture of processed cheese, disodium phosphate is added to give smoothness to the texture and to prevent fat separation.

distilled liquors A term generally applied to alcoholic beverages that have been distilled rather than fermented, although they may be distillation products of fermented beverages. Brandy is made by distilling wine, a fermented fruit juice, and rum is distilled from fermented molasses syrup. Whiskey, gin, and vodka are made from fermented grains, although vodka can also be made from potatoes. A distilled liquor contains about 170 calories per ounce of alcohol, but since considerably less alcohol is contained in a bottle of whiskey, vodka, or a similar liquor, 1 oz. of an 80-proof liquor contains only 65 calories.

distilled water Water that has been purged of minerals and other possible substances, including microorganisms, by distillation. Distilled water is theoretically pure water; it is used in scientific laboratory work in which it is important that the water be free of any substance that might distort crucial data. It has a flat taste and has limited use for human consumption because of its lack of minerals. Some bottled waters are distilled water with certain minerals added.

diuresis The increased excretion of urine, a process that is important in certain disorders marked by an excess of body fluid in the tissues, such as hypertension and congestive heart failure. Diuresis is also needed in the control of edema, which is characterized by tissues swollen from excess fluid. See *diuretic*.

diuretic An agent that increases the rate of urine excretion. Some common substances, such as caffeine beverages, aid in the excretion of urine. Various medications are prescribed as "water pills" to reduce fluid accumulation in the body by various methods. Some mercury-based diuretics reduce the ability of the kidneys to reabsorb water while cleaning the blood flowing through them. Others, such as the thiazides, work by increasing the body's loss of sodium and other minerals, which are associated with fluid retention.

diverticulitis An inflammation of the intestinal tract caused by irritation or infection of small blind pouches that develop in the lining and wall of the bowel. This condition commonly affects the colon and results from weak muscle walls of the bowel, complicated by chronic constipation. It is diagnosed with the help of a barium enema that outlines the diverticula, or pouches. Treatment includes bed rest, a bland or low-residue diet, cleansing enemas, and medications. In serious cases, surgery may be required to remove the affected portion of the intestine.

diverticulosis The presence of diverticula, or blind pouches, in the wall of the colon. When the diverticula become inflamed by bacteria or irritating substances trapped in the pouches, the condition is called *diverticulitis*. See this entry.

DMF Index The total number of decayed, missing, and filled teeth.

DNA An abbreviation for *deoxyribonucleic acid*. See this entry.

dolomite A mineral supplement that supplies both calcium and magnesium. The chemical name is *calcium magnesium carbonate*.

dopamine A neurotransmitter substance derived by the body's chemical processes from the essential amino acid *phenylalanine*. An enzyme in turn can convert dopamine into another neurotransmitter chemical, *norepinephrine*. Among the effects produced by dopamine are increased blood pressure and an increased rate of sodium excretion.

dose The amount of a substance administered at a given time to cause a particular reaction. Kinds of doses include a *curative dose*, which is the size of a dose needed to restore a patient to normal health; a *lethal dose*, or the amount required to kill a person; an LD_{50} dose, which is the amount of an agent that is likely to kill half the members of a population group; a *tolerance dose*, or the largest amount of a substance that can be consumed without causing ill effects; a *minimum lethal dose*, or the minimum size dose that will cause death; and a *divided dose*, or the fraction of a total daily dose administered at given intervals, such as once every four hours.

drops A method of administering vitamins to infants. However, drops are also used by older children and adults who have difficulty swallowing tablets or capsules, or who wish to measure their vitamins to a particular level. There are between 50 and 100 drops per teaspoonful, depending on the size of the drops.

dry milk powder Milk from which the fluid portion has been removed by spraying fine droplets of the skim or low-fat variety into a chamber through which hot air is circulated, or by allowing the milk to flow over two heated metal drums that rotate toward each other. Dried milk contains about 5 percent moisture, but more may be added to prevent clumping after it has been packaged. Dry milk powder has the same amount of protein, lactose, and minerals as regular milk and in the same proportions. However, it lacks the fat components as well as the fluid. One pound of nonfat dry milk powder is equivalent to 11 pt. of skim milk.

dummy See *placebo*.

dumping syndrome A condition that may occur in patients who have had surgery for partial removal of the stomach. It is characterized by weakness, dizziness, sweating, diarrhea, a sensation of warmth, or palpitation, or a combination of those symptoms. The condition may be controlled by a high-protein diet, taken mainly in small frequent feedings of dry foods, rest after larger meals, and medications. Partial stomach removal, or partial gastrectomy, is sometimes recommended in the treatment of peptic ulcers.

duodenal drainage test A test for the acidity of the contents of the duodenum, the first segment of the intestinal tract beyond the stomach, and for the presence of amylase and tripsin enzymes. The samples are obtained by stomach tube.

duodenal ulcer A peptic ulcer that occurs in the first couple of inches of the duodenum, near its connection with the stomach outlet. It is an ulceration of the mucous membrane lining the duodenum, in an area bathed by hydrochloric acid and pepsin from the gastric juices of the stomach. The most common form of peptic ulcer, the duodenal ulcer follows a pattern of symptoms. Pain, usually absent in early morning, develops in mid-morning. The pain is relieved by food, but returns an hour or so after a meal. A duodenal ulcer pain often comes at night, awakening the patient. The pain may also occur every day for weeks, then suddenly cease for a long period.

duodenum The first segment of the small intestine. It gets its name from the Latin word for "twelve" because the length of the duodenum is equivalent to the width of 12 fingers. It is the shortest but also the widest of the three segments of the small intestine. The pancreas, gall bladder, and liver secrete their digestive juices into the duodenum at a point about 1 in. from the pylorus, the valve through which the stomach contents empty partly digested food into the intestinal tract.

dynamic equilibrium A term used to describe the continuous tearing down and rebuilding of body tissues. The process involves much of the body, such as blood cells and skin cells, that are constantly being created to replace the cells that become worn out and are discarded. Even seemingly finished body structures like the skeleton undergo continuous changes with the removal and reorganization of mineral molecules. Protein molecules are also in a constant state of flux as amino acids are removed, reorganized, discarded, or converted to body fuel while being replaced by new amino acids in the diet.

dysentery A general term for a number of kinds of inflammation of the intestines, involving mainly the colon, with symptoms of abdominal pain, frequent bowel movements, the presence of blood and mucus in the stools, and painful or ineffective straining in an effort to empty the bowel. The cause may be protozoa, as in amebic dysentery, bacteria, viruses, parasitic worms, or chemical irritants. Dysentery caused by bacteria is the most common and violent form of the disorder and may result in as many as 40 bowel movements a day and a high fever. Dehydration is a common complication of dysentery because of the loss of body fluids in diarrhea.

dyspepsia See *indigestion*.

dysphagia A term used to identify any of several kinds of difficulty in swallowing. The person is usually aware of the problem and experiences a feeling that something is "stuck in the throat," a sensation that may or may not be painful. Some people have difficulty swallowing only solid foods and some experience dysphagia when ingesting both solids and liquids. The causes may be a disorder of the nervous system or of the muscles affecting control of the esophagus, or both, or a tumor or stricture in the esophagus.

dyspnea A medical term meaning shortness of breath. Dyspnea can be caused by a number of different conditions, including obstruction of the larynx, asthma, bronchitis, heart disease, a defect in the chest wall or lungs, or simply physical exertion. Dyspnea can also be caused by emotional disturbances.

dyssebacea A type of skin disorder associated with a deficiency of riboflavin and characterized by enlarged sebaceous follicles around the middle of the face. The sebaceous follicles are also involved in acne, but the disorders are not the same

e

ecgonine A substance related to cocaine that is present in coca leaves. Ecgonine has been reported to be present in small amounts in certain cola beverages.

eczema A type of skin inflammation marked by redness, small fluid-filled blisters that may ooze and crust, and itching. Eczema is associated with a wide variety of health conditions that are sometimes divided into two types of causes, exogenous causes, meaning external to the body, such as sunlight or contact with poisonous plants or chemicals, and endogenous causes, meaning internal causes, including such metabolic disorders as phenylketonuria or nutritional deficiencies like *pellagra*. See this entry.

edema Fluid accumulation that causes an abnormal swelling in body tissues. A common example is dependent edema, marked by puffiness that occurs around the ankles after a day of standing. Pitting edema is characterized by a persistent depression in affected body areas after pressure has been applied. Edema may result from conditions as varied as a physical injury or a nutritional problem, such as excessive sodium retention. Edema often is a sign of congestive heart failure.

edible portion The portion or parts of a food item that may be eaten after the inedible parts have been removed. The term has some importance for people on diets who must weigh their food accurately because of individual differences in what is considered edible or inedible. Some persons, for example, eat the skins or peelings of fruits and vegetables like apples and potatoes while others consider those parts inedible and discard them. Obviously, an apple that has been peeled and cored weighs less than a fresh, raw apple; there are also minor differences in caloric and nutritional values. A potato skin contains a significant percentage of the nutrients in a raw potato.

egg replacement value The extent to which a test protein offers the same nitrogen balance as a stated amount of egg protein used as the standard. See *nitrogen balance*.

elastin A rubbery form of protein found in the connective tissue of animals. Elastin is found primarily in food sources in the rump muscles of cattle. It is rich in amino acids and includes two amino acids not found in other tissues; however, because of its toughness elastin is not a popular source of nutrients.

electrocardiogram A recording made on a strip of paper of the electrical activity produced by the contraction of heart muscles. Although a heartbeat lasts only an instant, each stage of a contraction of a heart atrium or ventricle produces a particular tracing on an electrocardiogram. By examining the picture produced by the tracing, the doctor can tell whether heart function is normal. The electrical activity of the heart muscle is detected by electrodes placed on the chest and amplified thorugh a machine called an *electrocardiograph*. Abbreviated *ECG; EKG*.

electroencephalogram A recording on paper of the electrical activity of the brain cells. The electrical activity of the brain is detected by electrodes pasted to the scalp and amplified through an *electroencephalograph*. By examining the tracings, a medical specialist can learn much about the normal or abnormal functioning of a person's brain. For example, an electroencephalogram can help detect signs of a brain tumor, encephalitis, or different forms of epilepsy. Abbreviated: *EEG*.

electrolytes Substances that become ions when dissolved in a solution, such as a body fluid. Examples include sodium, chlorine, calcium, phosphorus, magnesium, and potassium. As electrolytes, the ions of those elements play an essential role in such body functions as contraction of muscle cells and the transmission of nerve impulses. The electrical qualities of these substances as electrolytes enable them to participate in the many electrochemical functions vital for normal cell life. Electrolytes also help maintain a normal balance of acids and bases, as well as fluids, in the body.

electrons Negatively charged particles of electricity that travel in orbits around the nucleus of an atom. The flow of electrons through a copper wire constitutes an electric current. When a radioactive element disintegrates, it may emit electrons as beta particles. Atoms sometimes transfer electrons or share electrons in chemical reactions, such as the formation of compounds. When an atom has a deficiency or an excess of electrons so that it becomes a charged particle itself, it is called an *ion*. See this entry.

electron transport chain A term used by nutrition scientists to describe the process by which electrons derived from food items in the digestive tract are transferred from one substance to another in various enzyme reactions. The chain usually ends in the final use of a nutrient by a cell when the electrical charge acts to combine oxygen and hydrogen in a molecule of water to be excreted.

element   The basic or primary part of something, a term that is usually applied to the chemical elements, which are the basic components of all matter. There are at least 105 chemical elements, each composed of a nucleus surrounded by a certain number of electrons orbiting about it. The composition of the nucleus and the pattern of orbiting electrons distinguishes one element from another.

elemental analysis   A description of a substance in terms of the chemical elements in its make-up and the proportions of the elements. The term may be applied to the entire human body or to a food item, such as milk, roast beef, or strawberries.

elemination diet   A system used to find an offending item that is the cause of a food allergy. The elimination diet consists simply of eliminating each of the food items regularly eaten, one after another, until one that appears to be the cause of symptoms is found. If the apparent culprit is singled out, it can be tested by adding it to the diet again and watching for adverse effects.

empty calories   A term sometimes applied by nutrition experts to food items that provide calories but few if any other important nutrients, like proteins, vitamins, or minerals. Foods that are rich in sugar, such as candies, are often cited as examples of empty-calorie foods. Another example is alcohol, which contains more calories per weight than sugar but has no other food value.

emulsifier   An agent that helps two normally nonmixable substances, such as oil and water, to be mixed. One example is the agent that allows oil and vinegar to be mixed in a salad dressing. Emulsifiers are commonly used in products like chocolate candy, in which it is important to prevent the cocoa butter from separating. A common emulsifier in many food products is lecithin, which is used in margarines and ice creams. Mono- and diglycerides are also employed as emulsifiers, and a substance known as polysorbate-60 serves as an emulsifier in puddings and pie fillings to keep the milk portion uniformly dispersed.

endemic goiter   See *goiter*.

endogenous   Anything that grows from or on the inside of a structure, such as the inside of a body organ or a tissue cell. The term is also applied to activities or processes that occur within the body and in some cases is used to indicate a trait or defect that is inborn or hereditary, such as an inborn error of metabolism. See *exogenous*.

endogenous carbohydrates Carbohydrates that are manufactured within the body tissues from proteins and fats. It has been estimated that about 10 percent of the fatty acids and nearly half of the amino acids in one's meals may be converted by the body to a simple sugar molecule, glucose, which is used as a source of energy.

endoplasmic reticulum A microscopic network of membrane tunnels that run through the cytoplasm of a tissue cell. They often contain ribonucleic acid (RNA) and function as miniature factories where protein molecules are built from amino acids.

endosperm One of the three main parts of a grain or seed of a cereal. For the benefit of the plant, it is the portion of the seed that provides nourishment for the sprouting embryo until the roots and leaves begin to function. The endosperm consists mainly of starch granules, although the outer portion, near the bran, may contain some protein. The bran and the germ are the other two basic parts of a cereal grain.

energy balance The balance between the calories consumed in food and the calories burned in physical activity. In order to maintain a constant body weight, caloric intake and caloric expenditure should be equal. One pound of fat is roughly equivalent to 3,500 calories. Thus, a person who accumulates an average of 10 calories per day more than the amount of calories burned should gain weight at a rate of 1 lb. per year. The body requires a certain number of calories per day as part of the basal metabolic needs, plus whatever amount of calories are required for an individual's work, recreation, or other activities. See *basal metabolic rate; calorie.*

enriched cereal products This term refers to cereal products, such as flour, bread, rice, and macaroni, to which thiamine, niacin, riboflavin, and iron have been added within the limits specified by the U.S. Food and Drug Administration. This is done to replace those nutrients lost in milling and processing. Certain levels of vitamin D and calcium are optional additions that, if used, must also be within a specified range.

enrichment standards The minimum and maximum amounts of each of the minerals and vitamins permitted to be added to a food under the regulations of the U.S. Food and Drug Administration.

enterogastrone A hormone produced by cells in the lining of the duodenum, the first segment of the small intestine. This hormone mediates the gastric activity of the stomach in response to the ingestion of fatty foods.

enteropathy A term used to identify any disorder of the intestine. This word is

enzymes

often accompanied by another term that describes the condition more specifically, such as *gluten enteropathy* or *protein-losing enteropathy*.

enzymes   A group of protein molecules capable of producing changes in substances necessary for life processes. Enzymes are involved in such functions as digestion, acid-base balance, and utilization of energy. An obstruction or malfunction of an enzyme system can result in an acute illness, leading to death or permanent damage, such as mental retardation.

Each enzyme has a specific role in life support activities and most have names that identify their role. Among digestive enzymes, for example, those that break proteins into amino acid components are called *proteases*; enzymes that break up fats are known as *lipases*, and starch splitters may be identified as *amylases*. A *transferase* is an enzyme that transfers atoms or ions from one molecule to another. *Oxidases* help respiratory activities and *carbohydrases* help metabolize carbohydrates.

Many inborn errors of metabolism and malabsorption syndromes may involve an enzyme deficiency. The complete metabolism of a food item usually requires a long series of steps and a different enzyme for each step; if one enzyme is missing, metabolism of the substance cannot continue and the residue of a partly metabolized food accumulates in the body tissues. One example is a disorder called *phenylketonuria* (PKU) that is caused by the lack of an enzyme with the long name of phenylalanine hydroxylase, which is needed to convert the amino acid phenylalanine into tyrosine, another amino acid. Phenylalanine accumulates in the blood and, if untreated, the condition results in serious damage to the skin, nervous system, and other organs.

epidemiology   The science of the relationships among various factors involved in the occurrence of diseases in the general population. An epidemiology study might be used to find a common factor among all the people in the United States who are afflicted with a particular disease, such as bladder cancer. The study would involve interviews with the patients to learn what sort of foods and beverages they consume, their ancestral background, the kinds of work they perform, life style habits like cigarette smoking, and similar information. Such a study might find that the common factor is cigarette smoking or coffee drinking, or both.

epidermis   The outer layer of skin, composed of a surface of dead cells covering a deeper portion of living cells. As new epidermal cells are produced in the deeper layer, the older cells die and are gradually pushed to the surface where they flake and drop from the body during bathing or from rubbing against clothing or other objects. The epidermis is about 1 mm. in thickness.

epinephrine   A hormone produced by the inner core of the adrenal glands, which rest on top of the kidneys. Epinephrine aids in certain functions of the nervous system. When a person is threatened, for example, the adrenal glands release epinephrine, which increases the blood pressure, the rate of the heart beat, the rate of breathing, and other bodily activities that are placed on an alert status to help the person cope with the threat. Also called *adrenaline*.

epithelial tissue Tissue cells that cover the internal and external surfaces of the body. The types of cells in epithelial tissue vary almost as widely as the surfaces in which they play a part, such as the enamel of teeth, the cornea of the eye, the skin, and the lining of the stomach and intestine.

Epsom salts See *magnesium sulfate*.

epulis The name of a tumor that may erupt from the gums, sometimes emerging between the teeth. The tumor is benign, that is, not cancerous, and may be associated with an infection in the area of the roots of the teeth. An epulis is easily removed by an oral surgeon.

equivalency A term used by doctors to indicate that two substances, such as a drug, are equivalent even though they are not exactly the same. For example, two substances that contain the same types and amounts of an active ingredient are called *chemically equivalent*. If the substances are absorbed and metabolized at the same rate, they are *biologically equivalent*. And if they have the same total effect on a person, they are *clinically equivalent*. See *niacin equivalent*.

ergocalciferol A form of vitamin D synthesized by irradiating ergosterol, a substance found in yeasts, fungi, and other plant life, with ultraviolet light. Also called vitamin D-2. See *vitamin D*.

ergotism A toxic condition resulting from eating rye or other cereal grains contaminated with a fungus of the genus *Claviceps*. This fungus, commonly called *ergot*, grows on grains and produces a mycotoxin that can be fatal when ingested by humans. In the Middle Ages this condition was called *St. Anthony's fire*. See this entry.

erythrocytes A word for red blood cells that combines two Greek words: *erythros*, meaning "red," and *kytos*, or "cell." See *blood cells*.

Escherichia coli One of the species of bacteria that normally inhabits the human intestine. Some strains of the bacteria are friendly and cause no problems, but a few wild strains of the species can be the cause of such disorders as diarrhea and urinary tract infections.

esophageal strictures A narrowing of the esophagus, or food tube to the stomach, caused by inflammation or ulceration of the lining of the esophagus. The strictures may also be the result of any of several diseases. The condition can be corrected by the use of devices that can be swallowed to widen the esophagus, then retrieved again.

esophageal varices A condition similar to that of varicose veins of the legs except that the dilated veins are in the esophagus and may be a cause of bleeding or discomfort in swallowing. The varices, or varicose veins, can be treated by surgery or the injection of drugs.

esophagitis Any inflammation of the lining of the esophagus. The causes may be highly seasoned or hot foods or beverages and also vomiting and hiatus hernia. See *hiatus hernia.*

essential amino acids Amino acids that must be contained in protein foods consumed by humans in order to maintain optimum health. In contrast to nonessential amino acids that can be manufactured by the body, the human mechanism is unable to produce the essential amino acids. They are: isoleucine, leucine, lysine, methionine, phenylalanine, threonine, tryptophan, and valine. Growing children also require arginine and histidine as essential amino acids; however, it is not certain that arginine and histidine are essential amino acids for adults.

essential fatty acid A fatty acid required for normal body functions that cannot be manufactured by the body and must be supplied in the diet. Only one fatty acid is truly essential. It is linoleic acid, which is found mainly in vegetable oils. Two other fatty acids are theoretically essential, but can be manufactured by the body tissues if other essential nutrients are included in the diet. They are linolenic and arachidonic acids. Also called *vitamin F.*

essential nutrients Any substance necessary for normal development and health maintenance that must be supplied by items in the diet. Examples of essential nutrients include the essential amino acids, essential fatty acids, and certain vitamins and minerals.

estimated intake Food intake estimated for the purpose of determining a diet, usually in terms of household measures rather than by weight or exact measurement.

estrogen A general term for a group of female sex hormones that may either be produced naturally in the body or manufactured synthetically. In the human body, estrogens are produced by the ovary, adrenal glands, testes, and placenta. Their functions include development of the secondary female sex characteristics and maintenance of an environment within the female body to sustain the life of an embryo.

ethical drugs   Another name for drugs that require a doctor's prescription. They are called ethical drugs because traditionally they are promoted only among members of the health professions and not to the general public.

ethylene gas   A gas applied to citrus fruits and bananas to increase their rate of ripening and color development. Without ethylene gas, bananas require about 1 week to ripen. Citrus fruits are placed in bins in which the atmosphere contains 1 part ethylene gas per 50,000 parts of air to develop full coloration.

excretion   The process of eliminating waste material from the body tissues. Excretion may include the loss of water and certain mineral salts through perspiration and the expulsion of carbon dioxide and water vapor through the lungs, as well as fecal excretion via the digestive tract and urine excretion through the kidneys. In addition to eliminating wastes, excretion is a mechanism for regulating the level of nutrients in the body. If, for example, the body's sodium content is high, sodium and water are excreted via the kidneys; if the level of glucose is high, glucose and water are excreted, and if the level of a water-soluble vitamin is excessive, it is also eliminated in the urine.

exogenous   Anything outside the body, including factors that may influence the body. One example is an air pollutant that may cause an attack of asthma. The opposite of exogenous is *endogenous*. See this entry.

exotoxins   Poisonous substances produced by bacteria but excreted by these organisms so the poison remains in the environment in which the bacteria lives or has lived. In some instances, food poisoning may occur because of the presence of an exotoxin that remains after the bacteria have been removed or destroyed. Botulism is an example of one type of exotoxin food poisoning.

extracellular   A term meaning outside the cell or cells. This word is commonly used to identify fluids, such as blood or lymph, that circulate outside the cell walls. Extracellular substances may also occur in various body spaces outside or beyond cell walls.

f

fabricated foods New and unique forms of food, or imitations of natural foods, that have been developed in a laboratory. Manufactured from ingredients obtained from agricultural products, fabricated foods are put together with the purpose of achieving predetermined characteristics, including nutritional qualities and how they look and taste. Margarine is a familiar example. Simulated meat made with soybean proteins is another.

fad diets Diets that are periodically popular as methods of rapid weight loss and that may or may not be variations of the simple rule-of-thumb that weight gain or loss is a matter of balancing caloric intake with calories burned by physical activity. Most fad diets appear to succeed because an initial effect can be the loss of several pounds of fluid from the tissues, after which the rate of weight loss slows considerably and is less impressive to the dieter. Fad diets usually result in a rebound effect, in which weight is gained back faster than it was lost. Also, most fad diets ignore the need for essential amino and fatty acids, vitamins, and minerals.

Fair Packaging and Labeling Act A federal law established in 1966 that regulates the advertising of foods and certain other products on radio and television and in magazines and newspapers.

FAO calorie standard The average minimum standards for calories and proteins established by the Food and Agricultural Organization of the United Nations. It is based on a theoretical man who is 25 years old, weighs 65 kg. (143 lb.), lives in a part of the world where the average annual temperature is 10°C (50°F), and works 8 hr. per day at a physically active job, requiring 3,200 calories in food intake daily. The standard woman is 25 years old, weighs 55 kg. (121 lb.), lives in the same climate, is either a housewife or a worker in light industry, and requires 2,300 calories daily.

fascia A type of connective tissue that resembles envelope-like sheaths that enclose other tissues. Muscles are enclosed in fascia sheaths, which produce their own lubricating fluid to reduce the friction of one muscle group rubbing against another.

fast foods Foods that can be obtained at establishments that specialize in carry-out meals available within minutes after ordering. This works by having the foods already prepared except for cooking or heating. Examples of fast foods include cheeseburgers, pizzas, french fries, chicken parts, and fish filets. Although fast foods tend to contain more fat and salt than necessary, some items, such as cheeseburgers and pizzas, can be adequate sources of the nutrients represented in the *basic food groups*. See this entry.

fasting To go without food and sometimes water for a set period of time. Some religious fasts specifically exclude water. After weight loss during a fast, the body tends to adjust itself by lowering the metabolic rate. Prolonged fasting can result in serious disturbance of body functions, leading to renal impairment, brain and nerve damage, and even death. As a means of losing weight, it should only be done under medical supervision.

fat content of diet The proportion of fats in the foods eaten daily. In North America, a typical daily diet supplies about 40 percent of total calories in fats. By contrast, in Japan a typical diet may supply as few as 10 percent to as much as 20 percent of calories in food fats. The American Heart Association has recommended that the fat content of the diet be restricted to no more than 35 percent of daily calories and with no more than 10 percent in the form of saturated fats.

fatigue The sensation of discomfort that occurs when energy output exceeds the body's restoration processes. Causative factors may include not only physical exertion and lack of sleep, but poor diet habits or emotional stress.

fats A group of substances formed by the joining of fatty acids with glycerin. Fats may range in consistency from light oils, such as olive oil, to solid tallows like deer fat. They are composed of large amounts of carbon and hydrogen and relatively small amounts of oxygen, a factor that makes fats particularly important as a source of body fuel; 1 g. of an average fat contains 9 calories of energy, or more than twice the energy available from an equal amount of pure sugar. Also, because fats pack more energy per measured weight than carbohydrates or proteins, the body is able to store more fuel in less body weight than would be possible if humans stored all their energy in the form of carbohydrates.

The average human body is between 15 and 25 percent fat. Thus, from slightly less than 25 lb. to more than 35 lb. of a normal adult's body weight is fat. At approximately 9 calories per gram, the amount of fat carried by a normal adult amounts to as much as 150,000 calories. If a person's body is 25 percent fat under normal conditions and he, or she, becomes 25 percent overweight, the amount of body fat in effect increases by 100 percent. This is particularly likely in later years when the proportion of fat to muscle normally increases and reduced physical activity tends to result in added body weight.

If it were not for other nutritional factors, such as maintaining a balance of protein, carbohydrates, vitamins, minerals, and water in the body, a person carrying 150,000 or more calories as body fat might be expected to live for more than 2 months without food, burning only the stored fat as body fuel. During periods of starvation, the body does use fat as a protein-sparing fuel. Fat deposits beneath the skin are usually consumed first, followed by metabolism of fat stores in deep body tissues. When a person gains excess weight, the storage areas beneath the skin are also the first to show the presence of fat. Since nearly all excess calories in the diet are converted to fat for storage, the body gains approximately 1 lb. of weight for every 3,500 calories consumed in excess of the calories burned in physical activity and the basal metabolic functions of breathing, blood circulation, and so on.

Human body fat is not an inert mass. Much of the adipose tissue of the body is in a constant state of being torn down and rebuilt. Because the free fatty acid components of stored, or depot, fat are quickly converted to body fuel, fatty acids are mobilized in response to almost any body activity, such as work, sports, sex, or even the body excitement stimulated by the mere act of watching a baseball or football game or a good TV show. The body's autonomic nervous sytem cannot tell the difference between watching a sports event or participating in a sports event or a fight for survival in a cave filled with saber-toothed tigers. When the primitive body instincts signal excitement, the bloodstream fills with molecules of fatty acids "shaved" from fat deposits and made ready as energy for body action. If the fatty acids are not required after all, the body's metabolic mechanism ships them back to the fat depots and puts them into storage again. The metabolic mechanism for fatty acid release is so sensitive, scientists have found, that simply eating a good meal or drinking a cup of strong coffee can result in fatty acids being released into the bloodstream.

In addition to serving as a source of body energy, fats provide a place for the body to store the fat-soluble vitamins, A, D, E, and K. Fats also serve as insulation and cushion material to help protect the skin and internal organs. Small amounts of fats are used in tissue cell structures.

Fats vary considerably in physical properties and digestibility. A fat that is liquid at room temperature is called an *oil*. Some fats that are solid at room temperature melt into oils at mildly warm temperatures. Examples include lard and butter. Mutton suet, however, has a very high melting point. Fats that are oils at room temperature are generally unsaturated fats, while saturated fats are usually solid at room temperatures, with a few exceptions. A saturated fat is technically one whose chemical bonds contain all the hydrogen atoms possible, so they are in effect saturated with hydrogen. When an oil is converted into a solid fat, as when a margarine is made from a vegetable oil, the process involves the addition of hydrogen atoms and the method is called *hydrogenation.*

A number of studies indicate that unsaturated fats, such as the vegetable oils, are more easily digested and are less likely to be a cause of atherosclerosis than the solid fats of butter and four-legged animals, red meats laced with fat. Beef and lamb fats contain about 50 percent saturated fatty acids, pork approximately 35 percent, and butter 55 percent, compared to less than 20 percent for most fish and vegetable oils. Exceptions include chocolate and coconut, two vegetable products with saturated fat contents exceeding those of beef and lamb fat.

Fat digestion takes place mainly in the small intestine where a pancreatic enzyme called *lipase* breaks the fats into glycerol and fatty acids. *Bile*, secreted by the gall bladder and emptied into the digestive tract, helps break large fat globules into smaller globules as food is churned by peristalsis of the intestine. Eventually, the fats are reduced to a very fine emulsion, called *chyle*, that can be absorbed by the cells lining the intestine.

Normal individuals can absorb about 95 percent of the fatty acids but persons with cystic fibrosis, liver disorders, malabsorption syndromes, and certain other diseases are unable to absorb fats adequately and much of the fat intake is excreted in feces. The digestibility and absorption of fats are also affected by their melting points. Butter, margarine, lard, vegetable oils, and meat fats with relatively low melting points can be digested efficiently in a normal digestive system. Besides the physiological benefits of fats mentioned previously, most fats enhance the acceptability of meals in several ways: They absorb other ingredients which add flavor and aroma to food and take longer to digest so that hunger for the next meal is delayed.

The proportion of fats in the diet seems to vary with the economic status of the eater. While most nutrition experts recommend that 20 to 25 percent of the total daily calories be in the form of fats, the average North American gets at least 40 percent of his daily calories in fats, but people in Third World countries often get less than 10 percent of their calories in fats. See also *fatty acids; essential fatty acid.*

fats and oils oxidation A process whereby oxygen atoms become attached to the molecular structures of unsaturated fatty acids, causing destructive changes. When an oily or fatty food becomes rancid, the cause is often due to oxidation.

fats and oils saturation The degree of saturation of the fatty acid components of fats or oils with hydrogen atoms. Generally, an unsaturated fatty acid molecule is able to hold more hydrogen atoms than it presently contains, whereas a saturated fatty acid contains all the hydrogen atoms possible in its molecules. An unsaturated fatty acid can be made to hold more hydrogen atoms by a process called *hydrogenation*, which is the method by which vegetable oils are converted to semisolid margarines.

fat-soluble vitamins   Vitamins that are soluble in fat or fat solvents and found in nature in fatty foods. This group includes vitamins A, D, E, and K. Fat-soluble vitamins taken in foods or supplements are stored in the body's fat deposits when they exceed daily requirements. As a result, deficiencies of fat-soluble vitamins because of an inadequate diet are unlikely. However, excessive doses of some fat-soluble vitamins, particularly A and D, can be harmful.

fatty acids   A group of about 40 organic compounds of a lipid nature found in plant and animal food fats. Nearly all of the food fatty acids are composed of carbon, hydrogen, and oxygen arranged in the same basic pattern that contains an even number of carbon atoms. They are generally classified as saturated if they have a full complement of hydrogen atoms, or unsaturated if they can accommodate additional hydrogen atoms in their molecules.

Saturated fatty acids with fewer than 10 carbon atoms are usually liquid at room temperature, while those with more than 10 carbon atoms are solids. Fatty acids from plants usually contain fewer than 16 carbon atoms whereas fatty acids from animals generally contain more. Fat from male animals usually has a higher proportion of saturated fatty acids than fat in female animals, a fact that applies to humans as well.

Humans utilize only about seven of the total number of fatty acids. This includes *lauric*, which comes from butterfat and coconut and palm oils; *myristic*, which is present in most plant and animal fats; *palmitic*, also found in most plant and animal fats; *palmitoleic*, supplied mainly by marine animal fats; *oleic*, generally available in plant and animal fats; *stearic*, mostly in animal but sometimes obtained from plant fats; and *linoleic*, found mainly in peanut, linseed, and cottonseed oils. An eighth fatty acid, *arachidonic*, found in animal fats, is present in small amounts in the human body and is essential for normal skin health. However, it can be synthesized by the body from linoleic acid, which is the only essential fatty acid normally required by humans. See *essential fatty acid*.

FDA   See *United States Food and Drug Administration*.

FD&C color   A color additive that has been certified by the U.S. Food and Drug Administration as safe for use in foods. The abbreviation, FD&C, stands for food, drug, and cosmetic. A law passed in 1960 authorized the government agency to identify as FD&C colors all food additives that had passed a series of animal tests for cancer, genetic defects, or other possible health hazards. An FD&C color is usually assigned a color name and number, such as FD&C Red No. 40, which is used in soft drinks, bakery products, candies, maraschino cherries, and many other food items.

Federal Food, Drug, and Cosmetic Act A U.S. government set of laws, first passed in 1938, that regulates the use of food additives, contamination of processed food by insects or other filth, and other health aspects of foods, drugs, and cosmetics.

Federal Trade Commission An agency of the U.S. government with responsibilities that include safeguarding the public by preventing false or deceptive advertisements of foods, drugs, cosmetics, or therapeutic devices, including the packaging and labeling of products. The Federal Trade Commission can demand the prosecution of persons responsible for false advertising of foods, drugs, and cosmetics that may be injurious to the health. Abbreviated *FTC*.

fermentation A natural process whereby certain strains of bacteria convert food elements from one form to another, as when grape juice is converted to wine or milk to yogurt. Many common foods are made possible by fermentation, including bread, cheese, sauerkraut, and soy sauce. Black tea is made by fermenting green tea leaves and coffee beans are extracted from coffee cherries with the help of a pulp fermentation step.

ferric chloride A compound of iron and chlorine used in medicine as an astringent and an antiseptic, and also in tests to determine whether a child has phenylketonuria (PKU). After a baby has been drinking milk for several days, a few drops of ferric chloride are placed on its wet diaper. If the baby has PKU, the urine spot will turn a deep bluish-green.

ferrous gluconate An iron compound that is one of the best sources of iron in the diet. Certain alternative iron compounds can damage the fat-soluble vitamins in the body. Ferrous gluconate is the form of iron commonly used in vitamin and mineral supplements.

ferrous sulfate A form of iron used in some medications to treat iron-deficiency anemia. Like ferrous gluconate, ferrous sulfate is regarded as less irritating to the gastrointestinal tract than other types of iron compounds.

fever blister See *cold sore*.

fiber A general term applied to cellulose, lignin, and other complex forms of carbohydrates that cannot be digested by humans. Some fibers are composed of chains of sugar molecules, similar to those in starch, but are connected in a way that cannot be broken down by the digestive enzymes in the human system. Other animals, such as cows, can digest fiber, which is why they can feed on grass and hay. However, the human digestive tract can use fiber because of the laxative effect of its bulk and because fiber binds water, which helps keep feces soft. Raw whole apples, peanuts, popcorn, whole-wheat bran, and broccoli flowers and stalks are good fiber sources.

fibrin An insoluble protein formed from a substance in the blood called *fibrinogen* during the blood-clotting process. During blood clotting, fibrin threads form a meshwork on which the rest of the clot develops.

fibroblast A type of body cell that is able to produce the fibers that become a part of the connective tissue. Fibroblasts usually develop special tasks in the body, such as producing fibers for bone, cartilage, or the collagen tissue of skin and tendons.

fibromyositis An inflammation of the fibromuscular tissue, which may involve ligaments, joints, or other limb structures.

fibrositis An inflammation of the muscle sheaths of the arms or legs. This condition is accompanied by pain and stiffness. The term is sometimes used by doctors to identify a problem commonly called *rheumatism*.

filled milk A milk substitute that contains skim milk and vegetable fats. Vegetable fats replace the butterfat, which is considered a rich source of exogenous cholesterol. Vegetable fats are generally unsaturated and less likely than butterfat to affect cholesterol levels.

filth tolerance The amounts of filth, such as insect fragments or rat hairs, allowed to remain in a given quantity of processed food sold to the public. For example, 100 g. (approximately 3.5 oz.) of peanut butter may contain 30 insect fragments and one rodent hair, while the same amount of broccoli can contain up to 60 insect fragments and still be considered safe to eat under a 1972 regulation of the U.S. government. While every effort is made to eliminate filth from processed foods, producing packaged foods entirely free of filth would become so expensive that consumers would not be able to afford them.

flatulence The excessive formation of gas in the digestive tract. Gas may result from swallowed air or from the fermentation of undigested food. Flatulence caused by bacterial fermentation can sometimes be controlled by reducing the proportions of fats, carbohydrates, and fiber in the diet. Although literally dozens of different foods, particularly beans, have been identified as causes of flatulence, there seem to be individual reactions to foods so that what causes flatulence in one person may not affect another.

flavin mononucleotide An alternative term for riboflavin phosphate, a coenzyme for a number of digestive enzyme functions. Abbreviated *FMN*.

flavoproteins A group of substances that are combinations of proteins and various forms of riboflavin (vitamin B-2). Recent research indicates that flavoproteins are involved in every major metabolic process of the human body as well as energy production. Flavoproteins are involved in the metabolism of other vitamins and enzyme systems. A deficiency of flavoproteins results in stunted growth and a variety of kinds of tissue damage and degeneration, particularly skin tissues. Flavoprotein deficiencies have also been associated with birth defects. The exact nature of the adverse effect depends on the kind of flavoprotein lacking in the diet.

fluoride A compound or ion of the element fluorine. One form of the substance, sodium fluoride, is sometimes added to milk, water, or juice as an alternative to the use of fluoridated public drinking water supplies as a protection against tooth cavities. Compounds of calcium fluoride or magnesium fluoride contribute to the development of hard bone tissue.

fluorine An element which is technically a gas but that also occurs in certain food sources as part of organic chemical compounds. Its main function in the human body is one of helping to maintain the structure and strength of bones and teeth. It is one of the more plentiful trace minerals, being present in the human body in amounts of 37 parts per million. A deficiency may produce symptoms of bone pain and a loss of calcium from the bones. Seafoods are a rich source of dietary fluorine, and it is added to the public water supplies of many communities. An excess of fluorine causes the appearance of black or brown spots on the teeth from mottling.

folacin See *folic acid*.

folate See *folic acid*.

folic acid A widely distributed vitamin of the B-complex. It is required by humans and many other animal species for normal growth and reproduction and as an agent in the formation of hemoglobin for red blood cells and the production of red blood cells in bone marrow.

Folic acid exists in several different forms and has certain specific functions in different animal species. In humans, folic acid is particularly important in the prevention of blood disorders. A disease known as *macrocytic anemia* occurs in humans deprived of folic acid. Other effects of folic acid deficiency include development of a smooth red tongue, gastrointestinal disorders, and diarrhea. Many animals are able to synthesize folic acid through bacteria in their intestinal tracts, but monkeys and humans are unable to perform this feat and must obtain the vitamin from foods in their diets.

Folic acid serves as a coenzyme for many bodily functions, including the synthesis of nucleic acids, which are necessary for the life of body cells, in the metabolism of most amino acids, and in the synthesis of certain amino acids. Folic acid molecules are also a source of carbon and hydrogen atoms needed by the body for the formation of other organic compounds vital to normal life functions. The name, folic acid, is derived from the Latin word *folium*, for "foliage," which suggests correctly that leafy vegetables are good sources of the vitamin. Other adequate sources are liver, yeast, and whole wheat. Also called *folate; folacin; vitamin M; vitamin B-c.*

Food Additive Amendment A law passed by the U.S. Congress in 1958 that defines food additives and requires that companies producing or using additives assume the responsibility for proving the safety of additive substances. The 1958 Food Additive Amendment includes the Delaney Clause, which forbids the use of additives found to cause cancer in laboratory animals. See *Delaney Clause.*

food analog A simulated food product that closely resembles a natural food in taste and function, but differs in structure and origin. One example is the low cholesterol egg analog, which is composed of vegetable oil, emulsifiers, milk solids, vitamins, and other additives. Also called *fabricated food*. See this entry.

Food and Nutrition Board of the National Research Council A branch of an independent agency of the U.S. government, located in Washington, D.C. Its functions include establishment of the *Recommended Dietary Allowances*. See this entry.

foodborne diseases Any health disorder caused by foods. Foodborne diseases include those caused by eating poisonous foods, such as rhubarb leaves; by chemicals, such as pesticides, sprayed on foods; or by disease organisms that infest foods, such as the bacteria that cause botulism or the small worms that cause trichinosis. Some individuals, because of genetic or other factors, may be more susceptible than others to certain poisonous foods; many types of seafood are deadly poisonous only at certain times of the year in particular localities. See *food poisoning.*

food-drug interaction A term that refers to the potential ill effects caused by reactions between foods and certain drugs prescribed or taken without prescription. One example of a drug that may produce adverse nutrition effects is the chlorthiazide type of diuretic, or "water pill," which can result in potassium and magnesium depletion. Alcohol, which may be taken as a beverage or as part of a medication, can interfere with body supplies of vitamins B-1, B-6, and folic acid.

food exchanges Commonly used foods grouped according to similarities in composition, so that those within a group may be used interchangeably in a diet. Diabetics use exchange lists, prepared jointly by the American Diabetic Association and the American Dietetic Association, as a food selection guide.

Similar lists have been prepared for reducing diets and other therapeutic diet plans.

food poisoning   A term used to identify any of a number of acute or chronic illnesses caused by eating foods that have been contaminated by poisonous substances or foods that contain natural substances that are poisonous to humans.

In some cases, food poisoning may be an allergic reaction or individual sensitivity to a food ingredient. Symptoms of food poisoning generally include an inflammation of the gastrointestinal tract, with tenderness, pain, and cramps in the abdominal region, nausea, vomiting, diarrhea, dizziness, and weakness. One type of food poisoning, however, the kind known as *botulism*, is more often characterized by visual defects, such as seeing double, headaches, constipation, difficulty in breathing and swallowing, caused by nerve paralysis. The most common form of food poisoning is caused by contamination of food by staphylococcus bacteria.

Quite often the contaminated food is one that contains cream or eggs, or both, such as custards, cream puffs, potato salad, or sauces, and has been allowed to remain exposed to the environment at room temperature. Many species of fish become poisonous as a result of feeding on marine organisms that contain toxins. This is especially true of tropical fish. However, at certain times of the year, other species also may be affected. Fish poisoning may also be caused by organisms that grow on the surface of the fish and are worked into the flesh by improper fish-cleaning methods. Ciguatera is a type of fish poisoning that has been known to cause death within 1 hr. Fava beans, also known as horse beans, cause severe reactions in persons who have not inherited the enzyme needed to metabolize the vegetable. Over 100 deaths occur each year from eating poisonous mushrooms. See *botulism*.

food processing   The system of preserving, storing, and remanufacturing food items so they may be available to the public throughout the year rather than only after the harvest season. Food processing includes canning, freezing, dehydrating, pickling, and other methods of extending the number of days or months that meats, fruits, and vegetables can be made available in a relatively fresh condition.

food satiation principle   A theory that certain cells in the hypothalamus gland regulate the urge to eat. When the amount of food needed by the body is consumed, a signal to stop eating is sent out. When this area is injured, it is known that an urge occurs to continue eating beyond the feeling of fullness. See *satiety center*.

food spoilage   The deterioration of the quality of food due to any of a variety of causes, including physical changes resulting from heat and humidity, chemical

food standards of identity

reactions among the food ingredients, the progressive action of enzymes that normally cause changes, and the infestation by insects, microorganisms, or animals like rodents.

food standards of identity   A term used by the U.S. Food and Drug Administration to cover packaged foods that are not required to list the ingredients on a label as long as the ingredients conform to certain standards identified with a particular food item. For example, a soft drink identified as a "cola" or "pepper" beverage is not required to state on the label that it contains caffeine, because caffeine is considered a standard ingredient of "cola" or "pepper" drinks. Similarly, a "jam" need not list its ingredients as long as it meets certain "jam" standards, such as the ratio of sugar to fruit.

fortification   The process of adding nutrients to foods, particularly to foods that naturally lack those nutrients. Examples include the addition of vitamins to cereals, milk, and margarine.

free radicals   A term applied to highly reactive fragments of molecules produced during metabolic processes, as in the splitting of a fatty acid molecule. Free radicals may react at random with damaging effects to other fats as well as proteins, vitamins, and enzymes. Free radicals are responsible for some of the unpleasant effects of rancid fats.

frenulum   A fold of membrane tissue that runs along the midline of the undersurface of the tongue and attaches the tongue to the floor of the mouth. When the frenulum is abnormally short, it can cause the condition known as "tongue-tie," or *ankyloglossia*. See this entry.

fructose   A sugar found in ripe fruits, molasses, syrups, and honey. It occurs in approximately equal proportions with glucose in oranges, grapes, and strawberries but in larger amounts than glucose in apples and pears. It has essentially the same chemical formula as glucose, with 6 carbon, 12 hydrogen, and 6 oxygen atoms, but with the atoms arranged in a different pattern. Also called *levulose*.

full liquid diet   A diet designed for use by persons suffering acute inflammatory disorders of the digestive tract, by patients recovering from surgery, and in the acute stages of many illnesses. As the name suggests, it is a completely liquid diet but it may include such items as cream soups and certain soft foods, such as ice cream and strained oatmeal.

functional ingredient   A food additive used for purposes not directly related to nutritional benefits. A functional ingredient may be one that improves the color, flavor, texture, or otherwise makes a food product more attractive to the consumer.

furry tongue   See *black tongue*.

g

GABA An acronym for gamma-aminobutyric acid, a neurotransmitter that plays an important role in the metabolism of substances within the brain cells.

galactose A simple sugar derived from lactose, or milk sugar. Galactose is also found in sugar beets, seaweeds, and gums, such as the mucilage of flaxseeds. In the human body, galactose is combined with a fatty acid compound found in tissues of the brain and nervous system. Galactose is also converted by the liver into glycogen, a body starch, for storage. See *lactase; lactose intolerance*.

galactosemia A genetic disease that requires treatment with a special diet based on restricted intake of dietary galactose. Because of an inability to metabolize the carbohydrate, galactose accumulates in the blood and urine, which leads to cataracts, jaundice, and mental retardation if left untreated.

gall bladder A small, pear-shaped pouch located just beneath the liver, where it serves as a storage space for bile produced by the liver. The gall bladder releases bile as needed for the emulsification of fats through a tube called the *cystic duct*, which joins another duct leading to the small intestine. An infection or disease involving the gall bladder, or the formation of gallstones, can interfere with its function.

garlic A bulbous plant, which, like chives, onions, and leeks, is a botanical cousin of the lily. Garlic has a pungent aroma that is desirable in certain food combinations, although much of the pungency is lost in wet cookery. Garlic is often used as a folk remedy by those who believe it has value as an antiseptic and antibiotic. Garlic oil obtained from crushing the cloves, or bulbs, of the plant is used to flavor a wide range of processed foods, including ice cream and candies.

gastric carcinoma A cancer of the stomach. It usually begins with symptoms of abdominal pain and indigestion, followed by loss of appetite and weight loss. Vomiting may occur frequently and the feces may show signs of bleeding,

gastritis A term for any inflammation of the stomach lining. The condition may be acute or chronic and can be caused by disease organisms, foods, beverages, or swallowed chemicals. The accidental swallowing of acids or caustic chemicals causes a condition known as *corrosive gastritis*. Alcoholic beverages and aspirin are common causes of *acute gastritis*. Symptoms may include loss of appetite, nausea, vomiting that may or may not be marked by traces of blood, and distress after eating. If the cause is a medication or something commonly consumed, such as alcohol, the symptoms usually subside when the culprit is no longer allowed to enter the stomach.

although blood traces are likely to appear as black in color rather than red because of the effects of digestive juices on the blood. The treatment for gastric carcinoma is usually surgery. The cancerous part of the stomach is removed and the remaining parts are stitched together to form a new, but somewhat smaller, stomach.

gene A self-reproducing unit of heredity located at a specific location on a particular chromosome. The unit is a segment of a DNA molecule. A chromosome may contain thousands of genes, each of which has a specific task in transmitting hereditary traits from one generation to the next. Genes generally contribute to the reproduction and development of offspring by controlling the synthesis of enzymes and proteins involved in building and operating body tissues.

generic drugs Drugs identified by their chemical or medical names rather than by brand names. The subject of generic drugs has been a source of controversy because although two substances may contain the same types and amounts of chemicals, one manufacturer may produce his product in a formulation that is more easily dissolved and absorbed than another, competing product.

geographic tongue A relatively harmless condition in which the surface of the tongue has bright red patches with light yellow fringes. The pattern can change from day to day as the discolored areas move to new and different parts of the tongue and the original red and yellow patches disappear from their previous locations.

geophagia The morbid compulsion to eat dirt; a form of *pica*. See this entry.

germ In cereal grains, the embryonic part of the seed. The nutrients in the germ often differ from those in the other parts of the cereal, the bran or outer covering and the endosperm, which is the portion outside the germ but inside the bran layer. Wheat germ, for example, is a rich source of thiamine and riboflavin as well as niacin and iron, while the endosperm is mainly a source of protein, niacin, and iron.

gibbed foods See *gibberellins*.

gibberellins A group of plant hormones that occur naturally in the seeds, roots, and young leaves of green plants. One member of the group, *gibberellic acid*, has been used to increase the size of tomatoes and other vegetables sold for human consumption. However, there is no evidence of harmful effects. Fruits and vegetables treated with gibberellic acid are sometimes referred to as gibbed foods.

gingivitis An inflammation of the gums, which doctors and dentists refer to as the *gingiva*. Gingivitis may take a number of forms, such as redness, swelling, bleeding, or ulceration. There may be changes in color or pigmentation of the area; a gray line along the gum margin is often a sign of lead poisoning.

glossitis An inflammation of the tongue that may be a sign of any of a number of health problems. The tongue may be swollen and tender, or it may simply have a burning sensation when spicy foods are eaten. An infection of the pharynx and scarlet fever are among possible causes of glossitis. Also called *red tongue*.

gluconeogenesis The process whereby the body synthesizes simple glucose sugar units from food sources that are not carbohydrates. Amino acids and fatty acids are the substances involved in gluconeogenesis. It has been estimated that the conversion of the amino acid alanine to glucose accounts for about half of the amino acid role in the process. Also called *glyconeogenesis*.

glucose A simple sugar that is the basic carbohydrate in many food products. It occurs in the blood and is the chief source of energy for most living organism functions. All digestible carbohydrates in the human diet are eventually converted to glucose during digestion. The rate of metabolism of glucose is controlled by the insulin in the body. Glucose that is not immediately required is converted to body starch, or glycogen, and stored in the liver and muscle cells. When the body runs out of places to store glycogen, the excess glucose is converted to body fat. Too much glucose in the blood is a sign of diabetes mellitus, hyperthyroidism, or hypopituitarism. Too little glucose results in hypoglycemia. See *diabetes mellitus; insulin*.

glucose-galactose malabsorption An unusual type of digestive disorder in which simple sugars like glucose and galactose cannot be absorbed through the walls of the intestine. Patients afflicted with this condition are restricted to carbohydrate foods containing fructose as a sugar.

glucose tolerance The ability of the body to utilize carbohydrates. A glucose tolerance test is employed to find abnormal carbohydrate metabolism problems in the body, such as diabetes mellitus or hypoglycemia. In a standard glucose tolerance test, a person is required to fast for a given period before being given 100 g. (3.5 oz.) of glucose. Then blood and urine samples are collected and analyzed several times over a period of 6 hr. Another type of test, called the *Exton and Rose test*, requires two 50-g. doses of glucose to be given 30 min. apart while blood and urine samples are taken 30 min. after each of the half-doses of glucose.

glucose tolerance factor See *chromium*.

glutamate A salt formed from the nonessential amino acid, *glutamic acid*. One example is monosodium glutamate (MSG). Glutamate can function as a neurotransmitter and can have either beneficial or detrimental effects on the central nervous system.

glutamic acid A nonessential amino acid widely distributed in proteins. Glutamic acid plays an important role in the excretion of ammonia, which would otherwise accumulate in the body with deadly effects. Glutamic acid obtained from vegetable protein is used in medicines for treating certain gastrointestinal and neurological disorders, and as a food additive to produce synthetic meat flavors, in salt substitutes, and as a flavoring for beer.

glycerin See *glycerol*.

glycerol A colorless syrupy liquid that has a sugar alcohol component, although it is derived from fats and oils. It is widely used in food manufacture as a humectant in candies and marshmallows, as an agent that gives body to gelatins, and as an edible coating for meats and cheeses. Glycerol is also used as an additive in a variety of products ranging from chewing gum to beverages. Some glycerol is produced as a by-product of wine making and may be included in sweet wines, which would be only slightly affected by its sweet taste. Also called *glycerin*.

glycine A nonessential amino acid that is a component of many proteins. In humans, it is involved in the formation of the hemoglobin portion of the red blood cell. Glycine is also used in medications administered as antacids and is included in dietary supplements. Also called *aminoacetic acid*.

glycogen A polysaccharide, or multiple-sugar-unit molecule, that is the form in which animals generally store excess carbohydrates. Glycogen is actually a starch that is formed by and stored in the liver. It is also stored in muscle tissue. When the body needs glucose in a hurry, it simply breaks up the glycogen chain of glucose units. The liver can store about 100 g. of glycogen and an additional 500 g. can be stored in the muscles. That amount represents approximately 1 day's reserve supply of glucose and it can be depleted by skipping a few meals. However, it is not wise to fully deplete the glycogen supply because a certain amount is needed by the liver for its functions.

glyconeogenesis   See *gluconeogenesis*.

goiter   An excessively enlarged thyroid gland caused by a lack of iodine in the diet that appears as a swelling about the neck. Goiter can also be caused by the use of certain drugs that block production of thyroid hormone by the gland. A goiter often develops during adolescence or pregnancy, when demands on the body's hormonal systems change. Treatment in most cases is simply an increased use of foods containing iodine, such as saltwater fish or iodized salt. Also called *endemic goiter*.

gold   The chemical element that is also a precious metal. It is usually present in the human body in an amount of 1 part per 10-million, or no more than 1 mg. To calculate your own worth in gold, divide the current market price by 30,000. Gold has no nutritional value but is used in some medications, particularly those administered for the treatment of arthritis. Otherwise, the body regards gold as a poison and various severe liver, kidney, and blood disorders can be caused by the presence of gold in the body tissues.

gout   A form of arthritis marked by joint inflammation, particularly at the ends of the arms and legs, such as fingers or toes, ankles, or wrists. The cause is an accumulation of uric acid crystals in the joints as a result of abnormal uric acid metabolism. Drugs and diet are used to relieve the pain and reduce the level of uric acid salts in the body fluids. An increased fluid intake often helps by keeping the uric acid salts dissolved; dehydration allows the crystals to settle out of the body fluids.

gram   A basic unit of weight in the metric system. There are approximately 30 g. per ounce. The word is derived from ancient Greek and Latin versions of *gramma*, meaning "a small weight." In the metric system, 1,000 g. equals 1 kg., which is equivalent to 2.2 lb. and 1/1,000 of 1 g. is 1 mg. Many of the essential nutrients are measured in milligrams. A standard helping of food is often given as 100 g., which is roughly equivalent to 3.5 oz.

gram calorie   A term for the small calorie used in measuring small amounts of energy, as in the metabolism of carbohydrates, fats, and proteins. A gram calorie technically is the amount of heat needed to raise the temperature of 1 g. of water by 1°C. Also called *gcal*. See *calorie; kilocalorie*.

GRAS   An abbreviation for *generally regarded as safe*, a term used by the U.S. Food and Drug Administration since 1958 to identify foods regarded as safe to use because of a lack of evidence that they might be harmful. Originally, all foods in use in 1958 that were not known to be dangerous when used in a normal manner were considered GRAS. In recent years, because of better scientific techniques and increased knowledge, many food items, such as caffeine, that were originally accepted as GRAS have undergone careful laboratory studies to determine whether they should continue on the government's official list of GRAS food substances.

gristle See *cartilage*.

gustatory A term that refers to the sense of taste. Taste buds that are sensitive to the basic kinds of taste are located on the inner walls of tiny depressions called *gustatory pores*, found on the surface of the tongue and sometimes on the epiglottis and soft palate.

gut An alternative term for the intestine, or bowel. The term is often used with a modifying word, as in *blind gut, catgut,* or *ribbon gut*. It is derived from an old Anglo-Saxon word for *channel* and is related to the word *gutter*.

h

hard water Water that contains an excess of minerals, such as calcium and magnesium. Hard water forms a scum with soap and results in scale deposits on metals. Hard water caused by calcium and magnesium is considered a temporary hardness because the minerals are separated from the water by boiling or other methods. Sulfur compounds can produce a permanent hardness that is not easily treated. A number of inconclusive studies have suggested that hard water provides some protection against heart disease whereas artificially softened water, which may add sodium to the diet, has the opposite effect.

health A state of physical and mental well-being, or the freedom from mental or physical disease or pain.

health food A term commonly applied to foods that are in a more or less natural condition and have not been treated with chemical additives or processed or manufactured in such a way as to alter the original nutrients. The term may also be interpreted to include foods grown without chemical fertilizers or pesticides, and natural food substances considered rich sources of particular nutrients. One example is seaweed, a natural source of iodine available to the public only through specialty stores. It should be noted, however, that all products sold in popular health food stores may not agree with the definition of health food.

heartburn A condition marked by a burning sensation in the lower esophagus, which may be felt in the chest area near the heart. Heartburn is actually a form of indigestion in which part of the stomach contents are regurgitated upward into the esophagus. The acid in the stomach's gastric juices then causes an irritating, painful discomfort. Heartburn may be secondary to another problem, such as hiatus hernia, an emotional upset, or improper eating habits. Also called *pyrosis*.

Heimlich maneuver A technique for treating a person who may be choking because of a foreign object obstructing the trachea. The rescuer stands behind the victim and places his arms around the victim's waist, allowing the upper portion of the patient's body to droop forward. The rescuer than makes a fist with one hand and places the other hand on top of the fist, which is positioned just below the victim's rib cage. The rescuer next presses the fist forcefully into the patient's abdomen with an upward thrust. The pressure of the fist should compress the lungs sufficiently to force the foreign object from the trachea. The procedure is repeated if necessary. Because a person with an obstructed trachea is unable to speak, the victim should use hand signals to inform companions or other persons nearby that he is choking. The Heimlich maneuver is also recommended as a preliminary measure to administering artificial respiration to a victim of drowning, electrocution, or other condition in which breathing has stopped. See *café coronary*.

heme   A compound of iron and an organic chemical called a *porphyrin*. Heme furnishes the red color and carries the oxygen in hemoglobin, found in red blood cells. See *hemoglobin; porphyrins*.

hemicellulose   A form of indigestible carbohydrate present in plant and vegetable food items. It is related to cellulose and other plant fibers that serve a purpose in providing bulk in the diet even though they offer the human no essential nutrients. Hemicelluloses are generally found in the cell walls of land plants. The corn husk is an example of a rich industrial source of hemicellulose that can be processed to obtain substances, such as gums.

hemoglobin   The oxygen-carrying red pigment of the red blood cell. Hemoglobin is composed principally of a protein, globin, and heme, a complex compound containing iron. Hemoglobin has the ability to combine with certain gases to form various substances like oxyhemoglobin, which is hemoglobin combined with oxygen from the lungs. Hemoglobin can also combine with toxic gases like carbon monoxide, which occurs in cases of carbon monoxide poisoning. Arterial blood is a brighter red than blood in the veins because it contains more oxygen. The function of hemoglobin is to carry oxygen to the body cells and transport carbon dioxide back to the lungs on the return trip of the blood circulation pattern.

hemorrhoids   A condition in which blood veins in the mucous membrane lining of the rectum become swollen and inflamed. The situation is similar to that of varicose veins, except that the location is the rectum rather than the legs. Symptoms include itching, pain, general discomfort, and often, bleeding. The cause may be pressure on the veins caused by straining to relieve constipation, pregnancy, tumor, or a circulatory disorder. Also called *piles*.

hesperidin   See *bioflavonoids*.

hiatus hernia   The protrusion of the top of the stomach through the diaphragm, a layer of muscle tissue that separates the chest contents from the abdominal contents. Several tubular structures, including the esophagus, normally extend through the diaphragm. The opening, called a *hiatus*, may be gradually widened by pressure of the stomach so that eventually a portion of the stomach becomes trapped in the lower part of the chest. Hiatus hernia is a common cause of heartburn symptoms.

high-calorie diet   A diet that provides upward of 4,000 calories per day, as may be required by some professional athletes and outdoor workers. Although a young mother may burn an average of 1,600 calories per day, studies show that on some busy days she may burn well over 4,000 calories. Olympic athletes frequently require diets providing 6,000 to 8,000 calories per day during competition periods. Studies of cross-country skiers show they may require as much as 9,000 calories per day.

high-carbohydrate diet   A diet that provides a great amount of calories in the form of carbohydrates. Carbohydrates are often increased in protein-restricted diets to contribute as much as 3,000 calories or more per day in order to spare protein metabolism by the body. The person on such a diet is encouraged to eat candies, honey, jams, jellies, breads, cookies, cereals, potatoes, and fruits.

high-fat diet   A diet that contains large amounts of fats. The diet may also be a low-carbohydrate, low-protein diet, as in a ketogenic diet, or one that simply contains large amounts of energy-rich fats in addition to normal amounts of carbohydrates and proteins. High-fat diets are utilized by persons who work vigorously in the outdoors, such as lumberjacks, who may burn thousands of calories daily from energy in fatty foods.

high-protein diet   A diet that contains two to three times the U.S. RDA levels of about 45 to 55 g. of protein per day for average adult men and women. A high-protein diet, for example, could provide an intake of as much as 150 g. of protein per day. High-protein diets are usually intended for people recovering from severe illness or injuries when it is important to provide amino acid building blocks so the body can build new tissues. High-protein diets are potentially harmful to the liver and kidneys and should be supervised by a physician.

high-sodium diet   A special diet for persons suffering from adrenocortical insufficiency (Addison's disease). Because the disease involves a deficiency of the hormone aldosterone, there is an increased rate of sodium excretion, resulting in a loss of normal electrolyte balance. The sodium excretion is accompanied by water excretion. In order to maintain normal electrolyte balance, the patient's meals must emphasize foods that contain large amounts of sodium or table salt.

hippuric acid A compound formed by the combination of the nonessential amino acid glycine and benzoic acid, a component of many fruits and vegetables. Hippuric acid occurs in the urine of most animals, but more commonly in the urine of herbivorous animals, or those that eat only plant materials. Hippuric acid production in humans is used as a measure of liver function. A liver function test consists of feeding a benzoic acid compound to a patient and measuring the amount of hippuric acid in his urine 4 hr. later. An abnormally small level of hippuric acid is a sign of a possible liver disorder.

histamine A substance present in tissue cells in all parts of the body. It is a product of the breakdown of histidine, an amino acid, and is usually released from the cells during antigen-antibody reactions, as in an allergic reaction to certain foods, hay fever pollen, or a mosquito bite. Histamine has the ability to stimulate the autonomic nervous system and circulatory system, causing some of the ill effects of an allergic reaction.

histidine An essential amino acid that is particularly important for the normal development of small children. It is also a precursor of histamine, which is present in all tissues and functions in a hormonal role. Folic acid is involved in the metabolism of histidine, and a folic acid deficiency is marked by the incomplete utilization of histidine. See *histamine*.

homeostasis The ability of an organism to maintain stability while adjusting to changing conditions in the environment. Homeostasis is necessary for a body to remain healthy or to recover from disease or injury. Foods and medicines play an important role in helping the body maintain homeostasis. Some homeostatic mechanisms of the body include keeping the body temperature at a steady level, maintaining an acid-base balance, and keeping up a steady flow of nutrients to the body cells while removing waste products before they can accumulate in the tissues.

homogenize The process of converting a mixture of materials into a substance that has a uniform consistency throughout. One example is homogenized milk, in which the cream has been thoroughly mixed into the rest of the milk by forcing it through special valves under high pressure; this breaks the cream globules into such fine particles that they cannot rise to the top, as would occur in normal milk and cream separation.

hormones Chemical compounds produced by one organ or gland and carried by the bloodstream to another organ or gland where they stimulate or retard a life process. Hormones are sometimes called *chemical transmitters* or *messengers*. In many instances, they have similar effects to those of nerve impulses, differing in that they travel in the blood rather than along nerve fibers. The total number of hormones in the body is unknown, but the adrenal glands alone produce more than 25 kinds. Each hormone has its own chemical formula and a specific function. One example of a hormone is insulin, which is produced by the pancreas but is carried to other body areas to help regulate carbohydrate metabolism.

hormones in food The hormones used to increase the rate of production of food items. One example is the hormone diethylstilbestrol, which is administered to livestock, particularly cattle, to speed up the rate of beef production. Plant hormones called *gibberellins* are sprayed on fruits and vegetables to increase the size of these products.

humectants Substances that act as moistening agents and may be added to foods to help maintain texture and other qualities associated with freshness. Glycerine, sorbitol, and mannitol are names of humectants used as food additives.

hunger A desire to eat that sometimes but not always is accompanied by physical sensations, such as hunger pangs caused by contractions of an empty stomach or a feeling of a need for energy. While hunger is generally assumed to result from food deprivation, certain psychological factors can also stimulate a desire to eat. One example is the sight or smell of food that stimulates the appetite when actually the body has not signaled a need for eating.

hydrochloric acid An acid formed by a combination of hydrogen and chlorine that occurs naturally in the gastric juices of humans and other animals. A deficiency of hydrochloric acid in the stomach, a condition called *achlorhydria*, is associated with stomach cancer, pellagra, pernicious anemia, chronic gastritis, and alcoholism. An excess of hydrochloric acid is called *hyperacidity* and is associated with emotional stress and tension and the formation of peptic ulcers. It is the hydrochloric acid of the stomach that causes the burning sensation of heartburn.

hydrocortisone A hormone secreted by the adrenal glands that is important in the treatment of arthritis because of its antiinflammatory action. Hydrocortisone is a glucocorticoid hormone, meaning it is involved in raising the concentration of blood sugar, as distinguished from mineralcorticoid hormones, which are associated with mineral metabolism. Also called *cortisol*.

hydrogen A chemical element that is a gas at room temperature when in a free state. It is a component of many vital life substances, such as water, hydrochloric acid, and the molecules of proteins, fats, and carbohydrates. The concentration of hydrogen ions determines the acidity of the blood and the acid-base balance of the body systems.

hydrogenation The process by which hydrogen atoms are added to fatty acids in order to convert a vegetable oil into a solid or semisolid margarine or shortening. The process requires adding hydrogen, which may be obtained from natural gas, to the vegetable oil in the presence of a catalyst of nickel or aluminum, or a combination of these metals. Hydrogenation is also used to make a special hard butter that is sometimes used as a coating for biscuits and other bakery products.

hydrogen ion concentration A term that refers to the acidity or alkalinity of a substance. The hydrogen ion concentration of a substance is indicated by the letters *pH*, usually followed by a number between 1 and 14. Pure water, which is neutral, has a pH of 7. Blood is very nearly the same number. If a pH, or hydrogen ion concentration, is less than 7, the substance is acidic; if more than 7, it is basic, or alkaline.

hydrolyzed vegetable protein A vegetable protein that has been broken down into its amino acid components for use as an additive in dehydrated soups, stews, gravy and sauce mixes, and also in canned chili and processed meats, such as frankfurters. Soybeans, which are about 40 percent protein and contain 18 amino acids, are often used as a source of hydrolyzed vegetable protein. Hydrolyzed vegetable proteins provide the nutritional equivalent of the original proteins and are often used in special diets for people who have difficulty digesting the usual food proteins. Abbreviated *HVP*.

hydroxyproline A nonessential amino acid present in proteins that form the collagen fibers of connective tissue. A type of mental retardation is associated with a disorder in which a person fails to inherit the gene needed to produce the enzyme that digests hydroxyproline; instead, the amino acid accumulates in the tissues in a condition known as *hydroxyprolinemia*.

hyperchlorhydria A condition of excess hydrochloric acid in the stomach, resulting in irritation of the stomach lining and general gastric discomfort. See *hydrochloric acid*.

hyperglycemia A condition of having an excess of blood sugar, or glucose, in the blood. Hyperglycemia can be a serious disorder, resulting in loss of consciousness and death in some cases. This condition may be associated with diabetes mellitus, with other pancreatic disorders, as a complication of burns, and with the excessive use of steroid medications. The high concentration of sugar in the blood draws water out of the body cells, resulting in a severe form of cellular dehydration. See *glucose; hypoglycemia*.

hyperphagia A medical term for morbid or pathological overeating. The condition may be caused by a disease, such as diabetes mellitus, or damage to the appetite control center in the hypothalamus portion of the brain.

hypervitaminosis An adverse health condition caused by consuming an excess of vitamins. The condition mainly involves excesses of the fat-soluble vitamins A, D, and K. Medical records show that overdoses of vitamin A have occurred among hunters eating the livers of bears and seals, which may contain millions of units of vitamin A. Overdoses have also occurred in infants administered doses too great for their body weight. Other cases have involved people who take vitamin A tablets for the treatment of sunburn. Chronic hypervitaminosis in adults usually does not develop until doses several times the recommended level are taken daily for a period of months.

hypoallergenic A substance that would ordinarily cause an allergic reaction but which has been treated or processed to reduce its allergic effect. When applied to cosmetics, hypoallergenic means that any known allergens have been eliminated from the formulation. Actually, according to dermatologists, allergic reactions to cosmetics are relatively rare and involve individual sensitivities to substances that may be in either hypoallergenic or regular cosmetics. See *hypoallergenic foods*.

hypoallergenic foods Foods that cause an allergic reaction when eaten, although the substances in the food fail to give a positive result in a routine allergy test. Almost any food can be hypoallergenic to one person or another, but the most common offenders are wheat, eggs, milk, seafoods, chocolate, strawberries, corn, nuts, and pork. One reason why a food may produce an allergic reaction in the digestive tract but fail to pass a skin test for allergies is that the food allergen may be altered in some way in preparing the extract for testing.

hypochlorhydria A deficiency of hydrochloric acid in the stomach. The condition results in difficulty digesting proteins and an increase in the rate of carbohydrate fermentation in the digestive tract. Bacterial action increases and diarrhea is a frequent complaint. It can often be controlled by increasing the intake of fruit juices and broth and restricting fried foods, cold foods, fats, and foods rich in sugar. Also called *achlorhydria*. See *hydrochloric acid; hyperchlorhydria*.

hypoglycemia A condition of having an abnormally low level of glucose in the blood. It can be caused by an overproduction of insulin by the pancreas, an excessive rate of consumption of blood sugar, or a defect in the secretion of glucose into the bloodstream. Symptoms may include mental confusion, hallucinations, convulsions, and loss of consciousness. Although it is not uncommon to experience a "low blood sugar" condition for a short period without ill effects, a true case of hypoglycemia can be serious and may involve tumors of the pancreas or other areas of the abdomen. See *glucose; hyperglycemia*.

hypovitaminosis A condition produced by the lack of any vitamin. Beriberi is an example of hypovitaminosis B-1 and pellagra is caused by hypovitaminosis B-3. Generally, any symptoms of hypovitaminosis can be treated by providing an adequate intake of the missing vitamin.

i

iatrogenic disease   A health condition caused unintentionally by something said or otherwise indicated by a doctor or other health professional. For example, a patient in otherwise normal health may become convinced that he has heart trouble because of questions asked by an examining physician, even though the physician never intended to suggest that the patient might have heart disease

idiopathic steatorrhea   A type of malabsorption disorder in which certain fatty acids cannot be absorbed and are excreted in the feces. People afflicted with this digestive disorder can obtain a special dietary form of fat manufactured from natural sources, such as butter and coconut oil, and combined with glycerol. This dietary product is known as *MCT*, which stands for *medium-chain triglyceride.*

ileitis   An inflammation of the ileum, the portion of the small intestine that joins the large intestine in the region of the appendix. The cause may be an infection, an obstruction, or a malabsorption disorder. Symptoms may include pain in the lower right side of the abdomen, or around the umbilicus, with loss of appetite, weight loss, anemia, and diarrhea that may alternate with constipation. Medications, special diets, and surgery are among types of treatments recommended.

ileocecal   The part of the intestinal tract where the small intestine empties its contents into the large intestine. The two parts of the intestinal tract are separated by an ileocecal valve that prevents the contents of the large intestine from backing up into the small intestine.

ileum   The part of the small intestine that extends from the jejunum to the connection with the large intestine. See *ileitis.*

impaction   The condition of being wedged firmly in a position that makes movement difficult. The term is often applied to a state of severe constipation, sometimes called *atonic constipation*, or "lazy" colon. Feces accumulate because of a lack of normal stimulus to cause a bowel movement. This condition is associated with abnormal eating habits, or lack of physical activity, or both, as may occur during a long illness.

inborn errors of metabolism Any of a large number of inherited disorders characterized by the lack of an enzyme needed for a step in food metabolism or a defect in protein molecule structure that interferes with normal metabolism. Many inborn errors involve an inability of the body to handle one or more of the amino acids. The general pattern of this disorder is one in which the lack of an enzyme blocks the complete metabolism of the amino acid. The amino acid or a by-product of its metabolism accumulates in the body tissues, causing mental retardation, atrophy of the muscles, bone abnormalities, or some other health problem. Treatment generally requires a special diet.

incomplete protein Any protein that lacks one or more of the essential amino acids and is incapable of supporting life. Incomplete proteins are generally found in foods of plant origin, such as legumes, grains, and nuts, whereas foods of animal origin, particularly eggs, milk, and cheese, are sources of complete proteins.

index of nutritional quality A system of organizing information about various food items to show the proportions of important nutrients as compared to their caloric content per serving. The index can also be used to plan combinations of complementary foods so that meals include food items with more of the essential nutrients, which might otherwise be overlooked. Also called *nutrient density*.

indigenous Something that is native to a particular place. One example is coffee, which is indigenous to Ethiopia, where it originated, although it is now grown in tropical regions throughout the world. Many North American herbs are indigenous to Europe but were transplanted by settlers of the original colonies.

indigestion A word literally meaning an "absence or failure of normal digestion." The term is commonly used to describe any vague discomfort of the abdominal area following a meal, with symptoms of flatulence, heartburn, nausea, cramps, belching, vomiting, or diarrhea. Ordinary indigestion is often caused by eating too much, eating too fast, eating food that is too fatty or spicy or poorly prepared, or by emotional stress or anxiety. It can also be caused by serious problems, like food poisoning, peptic ulcer, gall bladder inflammation, food allergy, appendicitis, an infectious disease, such as influenza, or a heart attack.

infant nutrition The special dietary needs of children during the first 2 years or so after birth. The normal infant requires an average of about 50 calories per day per pound of body weight and a relatively high fluid intake. During early infancy, the protein and fat content of breast milk is appropriate for the child's needs of those food elements. Cow's milk may provide more calcium and phosphorus than breast milk, but either type of milk may require vitamin supplements, particularly vitamins A, C, D, thiamine, niacin, and riboflavin. The infant's need for amino and fatty acids and vitamins and minerals should be met before carbohydrates are added for satiety's sake.

infarction An area of dead tissue caused by an arterial obstruction that cuts off the supply of fresh blood to the area. A myocardial infarction is one that involves heart muscle damage caused by a blocked artery. An infarction of the intestine can be caused by a hernia that interrupts blood flow to a segment of the bowel.

infection Any disease condition produced by the invasion of body tissues by microorganisms. The microorganisms may be viruses, bacteria, fungi, protozoa, tiny worms called *nematodes*, or organisms called *rickettsiales*, which resemble a cross between viruses and bacteria. An infection can be acquired by eating contaminated food or drinking contaminated beverages, from inhaling disease agents in tiny fluid droplets or dust particles, through a wound or break in the skin or a mucous membrane, by a blood transfusion or organ transplant from an infected donor, by person-to-person contact, or by indirect contact by using a towel, clothing or other item previously used by an infected person. Infections have occurred by using a borrowed lipstick, by scratching a bug bite, and by breathing air from a contaminated air conditioner. Specific symptoms vary with the particular type of disease organism and the method of body invasion, but infections usually have in common a form of inflammation that results when the body's immune system releases its antibodies to resist the invasion. Treatment also varies with the type of disease organism; even among bacteria-fighting medications, there are specific types of antibiotics for certain kinds of germs.

influenza An acute respiratory disease caused by a virus and characterized by symptoms of fever, coughing, headache, inflammation of the breathing passages, and a general feeling of illness. There are three basic types of influenza virus, identified as Types A, B, and C, and numerous strains of each type. Type A influenza is the most common form of the disease, and is usually spread by person-to-person contact and inhalation of air-borne droplets. Acute epidemics of influenza occur in North America about once every 3 years during early winter. Outbreaks of Type B influenza occur about once every 5 years. Type C influenza is usually not a cause of epidemics.

ingestion The act of taking something into the mouth, such as food or medicine. The term is also used to describe the swallowing of toxic materials, such as poisons or drugs of abuse. It is derived from a Latin word *ingestus*, which means "to carry in."

inorganic compounds A term that generally refers to any chemical compound which does not contain carbon. The division between organic and inorganic chemicals is not sharp. Many substances occur in nature with carbon as an element even though they have nothing to do with living organisms, which is the basis for the distinction. Sometimes inorganic compounds are further defined as chemical compounds lacking both carbon and hydrogen.

inositol A sugar-like vitamin of the B-complex present in many plant and animal tissues as well as some microorganisms, such as yeast cells. Inositol is involved in the metabolism of carbohydrates and fats and is considered essential in human nutrition. In animal experiments, inositol has been found to protect against fatty liver and alopecia, a type of baldness. Inositol is also a precursor of phytic acid, a substance in certain plant sources of food that binds calcium, iron, and magnesium so they cannot be absorbed from the walls of the small intestine.

inpatient A person who has been admitted to a hospital or other health facility as a temporary resident, even though it may only be for an overnight stay. A patient who lives at home but makes a trip to a hospital, clinic, or other facility for treatment during the day is called an *outpatient*.

insecticides Chemical agents that kill insects. Most commercial insecticides are potentially harmful to humans. Insecticides are usually designed for a particular purpose, such as *stomach insecticides*, which are used to control chewing insects like caterpillars. *Contact insecticides* are used against insects that have a cuticle, or hard outer surface. *Fumigant insecticides* are designed to be inhaled by insects. *Biodegradable insecticides* are broken down sooner or later into harmless residues, but some synthetic compounds, such as those containing ethylene dibromide (EDB), are intended to resist breaking down and are more likely to enter the food supply or prove harmful to birds, fish, and other animal life.

insulin A hormone secreted by the pancreas into the blood where it regulates the metabolism of carbohydrates, amino acids, and fatty acids. Because insulin is necessary for the prevention of diabetes mellitus, it is sometimes called the *antidiabetic factor*. Insulin is essential for normal life because it enables the liver to store glucose, the basic sugar molecule derived from the metabolism of carbohydrates. When insulin is lacking in the bloodstream, the excess sugar, which cannot be stored as glycogen, spills over into the urine. When carbohydrates cannot be metabolized normally because of a lack of insulin, fatty acids and amino acids are not properly metabolized either.

insulin shock An adverse effect of an insulin overdose or an inadequate food intake with a normal dose of insulin. The condition affects diabetes mellitus patients whose meals are delayed or irregular, or as a result of physical exertion that burns glucose in the blood more rapidly than expected. Symptoms include extreme hunger, cold sweats, tremors, dizziness, nausea, weakness, and drowsiness. If not controlled, the condition progresses to convulsions, muscle spasms, and unconsciousness. Insulin shock is easily treated by giving the victim candy, sweetened orange juice, or some other sugar-rich food at the first signs of shock.

intake An alternative term for ingestion, but often used with a modifying term pertaining to the size of the dose or serving ingested, such as an intake of 100 g. of glucose

internal medicine A medical specialty that is generally concerned with diseases that do not require surgery. Problems of the digestive tract, for example, may be treated by a specialist in internal medicine. When surgery is required, the internist—a title sometimes used to identify an internal medicine specialist—usually works with the surgeon as needed before and after the operation.

international unit A standard of measurement of the amount of a pure vitamin needed to produce an effect in an animal. For example, 1 IU of vitamin C is equal to 0.05 mg. or 50 mg. of pure ascorbic acid. A certain number of international units of vitamin C is required to prevent or cure scurvy symptoms in a species. The international units, which are not always used for all vitamins, were established because of confusion about the amount of a vitamin recommended or required for normal health. Abbreviated *IU*.

intestinal flora A polite term for the bacteria that normally flourish in a person's intestinal tract. In addition to a variety of strains of bacteria, the intestine is home to a number of yeasts and molds. The types of microorganisms vary somewhat from one person to another, depending on the amounts of carbohydrates and proteins they eat; carbohydrates attract one kind and proteins another. The intestine of a newborn infant is sterile, but it soon begins to acquire microorganisms from either breast milk or cow's milk. Intestinal flora are important in helping the body synthesize vitamins B-12, K, thiamine, biotin, folic acid, and possibly niacin.

intoxication The term literally means "a state of being poisoned," as a toxic substance is a poison. The word is commonly used to describe the adverse effects of alcohol, which is a toxic substance. However, an excess amount of a great number of substances can produce symptoms of intoxication. Acidosis and alkalosis are examples of intoxication. An allergic reaction can also be a form of intoxication. See *water intoxication*.

intravenous The injection of a substance into a blood vein. Intravenous feeding is often a method used of providing fluids with or without nutrients when a person is suffering from severe dehydration or is unable to drink fluids for various reasons, such as surgery for an abdominal problem. Intravenous feeding is also used to provide nourishment for an unconscious person. Because drugs are also administered by intravenous methods, hospital personnel must be cautious about food and drug interactions since medications and nutrients may drip into the same vein.

intrinsic factor A protein substance secreted by glands in the stomach that is necessary for the absorption of the vitamin B-12 *extrinsic factor*, sometimes called *cyanocobalamin*. Absorption of the extrinsic factor is necessary to prevent pernicious anemia. A failure of the stomach glands to produce the intrinsic factor is a chief cause of pernicious anemia.

invert sugar A mixture of dextrose and levulose sugar molecules obtained by splitting sucrose molecules. The half-and-half mixture of sugars is sweeter than plain sucrose and does not crystallize as easily, factors that make invert sugar a popular item for food processors. Invert sugar is made by exposing sucrose to an acid or an enzyme, invertase. It also occurs naturally in the form of honey, which is approximately one-half dextrose (glucose) and one-half levulose (fructose).

iodine A mineral that is essential for normal human health because it is involved in the formation of thyroid hormone, which in turn controls the metabolic rate of the individual. Iodine is also distinguished by the fact that a deficiency of the mineral in the soil produces its effects in the physical appearance of persons who eat foods grown in that deficient soil. The thyroid hormone is secreted by the thyroid gland, which works overtime when iodine is lacking in food to compensate for the absence of the mineral. The overactivity of the gland, which is located in the neck, causes the gland tissues to become enlarged, resulting in a huge swelling, called a *goiter*, in the person's neck.

With a few exceptions, iodine-deficient soil occurs mainly in areas located in inland geographic regions, or away from oceans, which are a main iodine source. One exception is Japan, which has iodine-poor soil, yet the traditional diet of the Japanese is rich in seafoods, including seaweed. In the United States and other parts of the world, the major source of iodine is iodized salt, which is ordinary table salt to which potassium iodide has been added during processing on the assumption that if enough table salt is added to one's food iodine deficiency will not develop. Other types of iodine supplements are available for people on low-sodium diets who cannot add table salt to their food. Iodine deficiency is particularly critical for pregnant women, nursing mothers, and adolescents, who have much greater-than-average needs for iodine. A thryoid-deficient mother may deliver a physically and mentally retarded child. See *iodized salt*.

iodized salt Table salt (sodium chloride) that contains a small amount of potassium iodide. Potassium iodide is added to assure the general public of a source of the essential nutrient iodine in their meals. Only a very small amount of potassium iodide, about 1/100 of 1 percent, is added to table salt, but it is enough to provide about twice the required amount of iodine for the average adult, who uses about 6 g. of table salt daily in his food. The iodine is needed for normal functioning of the human thyroid gland. See *goiter; iodine; table salt*.

iodopsin A photochemical pigment found in the retina of the eye. It is a chemical complex of vitamin A and a protein and is important for color vision. Also called *visual violet*.

ion An atom or group of atoms carrying an electrical charge. The electrical charge, which may be either negative or positive according to the atomic nature of the ion, influences the manner in which it will react with other ions or substances. Ions in body tissues or fluids are called *electrolytes*. See this entry.

iron A mineral required by the body for the production of hemoglobin and myoglobin molecules, the iron-protein complexes that allow red blood cells to carry oxygen from the lungs to the various body tissues. They are also the means of storing a few minutes' worth of emergency oxygen supply in the muscle tissues.

The hemoglobin molecule makes it possible for blood to carry 60 times as much oxygen as would be possible if the body had to depend on the amount of oxygen that could be dissolved in the blood's fluid. Hemoglobin also carries carbon dioxide waste gas from the body tissues to the lungs, to be exhaled. It sometimes unwittingly attracts toxic substances, such as carbon monoxide molecules, which render blood cells useless so they must be replaced. Iron is one of the more abundant trace minerals in the body; the average adult body contains about 65 parts per million of iron. The average adult also needs about 10 mg. of iron daily to replace losses; growing children and pregnant or menstruating women need up to 20 mg. per day. Menstruating women and people with blood losses from ulcers or other diseases or injuries may develop iron-deficient anemia when the mineral is not replaced as fast as it leaves the body.

The body usually absorbs only a portion of the iron in the diet, apparently taking in what is absorbable; some iron compounds cannot be absorbed through the intestinal walls. Iron from animal food sources is absorbed more easily than iron from plant sources, which is better absorbed when eaten with meats than in a purely vegetarian diet. Meats and organ meats, such as liver, are the animal food sources. Leafy vegetables, legumes, and dried fruits are among the better vegetarian sources. Molasses is a relatively good source of iron.

An excess of iron can be just as dangerous as a deficiency of iron. Although vitamin C increases the body's ability to absorb iron, too much iron causes the body to lose its vitamin C so that symptoms of scurvy may develop. Because excess iron is stored in the liver, liver damage is a common adverse effect. Iron can also damage the pancreas, increasing a person's susceptibility to diabetes. A type of bone softening that involves the lower back is still another adverse effect of too much iron in the diet.

iron-deficiency anemia   A form of anemia characterized by an inadequate amount of iron in the body stores, a low level of iron in the blood, or a low concentration of hemoglobin in the red blood cells. The average adult requires about 15 mg. of new iron every day, but growing children and menstruating women often require a greater proportion per body weight. Iron deficiency often occurs in children who depend on milk as a main source of nutrients since milk is a poor source of iron. Muscle and organ meats are the best sources. Worldwide, iron deficiency is the most common cause of anemia.

irradiation   The act of exposing something to radiant energy. Although irradiation commonly refers to the use of radioactive materials, it can also mean the application of heat or sunlight, x-rays, cosmic rays, infrared, or ultraviolet radiation. Irradiation is used in the diagnosis and treatment of physical disorders and in the preservation of food, since radiant energy can destroy bacteria and other microorganisms that ordinarily cause food spoilage.

irritable colon syndrome   See *colitis*.

ischemia   A medical term that means blood starvation, or oxygen starvation of tissues that cannot get an adequate supply of oxygen-rich blood. Ischemia of the heart can produce painful symptoms of a heart attack; ischemia of the brain results in a stroke. The cause of blood deficiency is usually a blocked artery or a constricted artery. The word ischemia is derived from two Greek terms, *ischein*, meaning "to suppress," and *haima*, meaning "blood."

isolate   A term that means something that has been separated in pure form from a complex mixture of substances. If pure vitamin C could be separated from the other substances in orange juice, it would be an isolate.

isoleucine One of the essential amino acids. It is found in fibrin and other proteins and is required for normal infant growth and for nitrogen balance in adults. The sources of isoleucine are milk, eggs, and meats. Lesser amounts are available from vegetable food sources.

isometrics A system of exercise and muscle development in which muscle tension is increased against resistance, although there is no movement at the neighboring joints. See *isotonics*.

isotonics A system of physical exercise in which the muscles are contracted, although muscle tension does not change during the activity. The muscle shortens during contraction, although the load on it remains the same. See *isometrics*.

j

jaundice A discoloration of the skin caused by an accumulation of bile pigments in the bloodstream. The bile pigment produces a yellow coloration in the skin and the normally white areas of the eyes. The discoloration is often not noticeable in artificial light, but may be obvious when the person is exposed to sunlight. The bile pigment, known by the medical name of *bilirubin*, is a by-product of the breakdown of old red blood cells. Ordinarily, bile waste products are excreted in the feces or urine, but in the case of a gall bladder or liver disorder, such as hepatitis, the pigment accumulates in the blood and is circulated to the various body tissues.

jejunum The middle section of the small intestine. The jejunum is about 8 ft. long and is lined with numerous folds of mucous membrane covered in turn with a carpeting of velvet-like villi. The villi, tiny projections into the interior of the intestine, contain blood and lymph vessels that carry away nutrients absorbed from the food being digested. The membrane folds and villi increase by many times the amount of intestinal wall lining that can be exposed to the digesting food passing through the jejunum.

jogging A form of aerobic exercise that requires a significant increase in calorie burning and breathing rate, compared to an exercise like walking. Jogging at a pace of 6 mph utilizes 3 to 4 times as much oxygen as walking over the same terrain at 3 mph. It also requires between 25 and 30 more calories of energy per mile than walking. Jogging is performed as a type of trotting at a steady, measured pace, as distinguished from running, as in a footrace.

joule A unit of energy measure sometimes used by nutrition experts and other scientists. It is roughly equivalent to 4.2 calories.

junk food A popular term applied to food items that are attractive in terms of sweetness, colorings, and flavorings, but which have little or no nutritional value other than calories. A junk food item is generally rich in sugar, flour, and fats, and is manufactured with appropriate additives to give it texture, body, and other characteristics that appeal to the appetite-stimulating sensory organs of the body.

k

Karell diet A diet used in the treatment of congestive heart failure and kidney inflammation. It consists of nearly 1 qt. of milk daily, usually skim milk, for 1 week, followed by the gradual addition of eggs, dry toast, meat, rice, and vegetables. It was developed by a nineteenth-century physician, Philip Jakob Karell.

kelp A type of seaweed that has been used since ancient times as a goiter preventive. Kelp, which grows in deep, rocky ocean areas, is rich in iodine, the mineral that prevents goiter, a sign of thyroid gland dysfunction. It reportedly contains about 20 amino acids and varying amounts of numerous minerals and vitamins, including vitamin B-12, which rarely occurs in plant food sources. References to the use of kelp are found in writings of ancient Greek and Chinese physicians, but the value of the seaweed was not discovered until the seventeenth century by the Japanese, who now make extensive use of kelp and other seaweeds in their meals.

Kempner's rice-fruit diet A rice diet introduced in 1944 by American physician Walter Kempner for people with high blood pressure (hypertension) and kidney disease. It consists of rice and fruit or fruit juices, plus sugar, iron, and vitamins. Meals are prepared from a daily ration of 8 to 12 oz. of rice, cooked or steamed, without salt, milk, or fat added. The diet limits sodium intake to less than 150 mg. daily. See *rice diet*.

keratin A tough protein substance manufactured by the cells of the epidermis. The horny layers of the epidermis, as well as the hair and skin, contain large amounts of keratin. Although hard when dry, keratin is softened by water and certain chemicals, which makes it possible to fashion a hair style when the hair is warm and moist.

keto acid One of the first substances formed by the metabolism of an amino acid. Keto acids are also produced by the metabolism of fatty acids. They are carried by the bloodstream to various body tissues where they participate in the metabolism of carbohydrates and are themselves eventually converted to carbon dioxide and water.

ketogenic diet   A diet that contains large amounts of fats, with small amounts of proteins and carbohydrates. A ketogenic diet may be prescribed to produce a condition of ketosis and has been used in the treatment of epilepsy in children. See *ketosis*.

ketone bodies   The term used to identify certain by-products of the metabolism of fatty acids which are utilized by muscle tissue. One example of a ketone body is acetone. Under normal conditions, ketone bodies are broken down into carbon dioxide and water by the liver and other tissues. Also called *acetone bodies*.

ketosis   An excessive increase of ketone bodies in the bloodstream and tissues resulting from incomplete oxidation of fatty acids. This elevated level upsets the body's acid-base balance, which may lead to severe acidosis. The initial cause is the lack of carbohydrates in the diet or the improper utilization of carbohydrates as can occur in a disease, such as diabetes mellitus. A sign of ketosis is what is called a sweet or fruity breath.

kidney   Two bean-shaped organs, each about 4 in. long and 2 in. wide, located in the abdomen between the top of the pelvis and the bottom of the rib cage. Their function is to filter the blood, excrete the waste products of cellular metabolism, and regulate the concentrations of water and electrolytes in the body fluids. The dissolved waste products and excess fluid are excreted as urine.

Each kidney contains about 1 million tiny filters called *nephrons* that have the job of literally taking the blood apart and putting it back together again. Each drop of blood goes through this filtering process several times a day. It has been calculated that the kidneys filter the equivalent of the body's entire fluid content every 6 hr. They receive up to 25 percent of all the blood pumped by the heart every minute. However, they release only about 1 percent of the fluid received, yet it amounts to more than 1 qt. of urine daily.

Blood enters the kidney through an artery, the *renal artery*, and is diverted into one of the nephron units. The filtration process is aided by fluid pressure as blood cells, water, dissolved minerals, and other substances are separated, sorted, and either routed into the urinary tract or put back into the bloodstream that flows from the kidney via a renal vein. How the kidneys decide which parts of the blood to keep and which parts to throw away in the urine is something of a mystery. However, it is known that various organ systems send messages to the kidneys advising them, for example, to save potassium today or dump the potassium because the body has all it needs.

kidney stones Stones that form in the kidneys when the concentration of solids in the urine is too great for the amount of fluid. The stones form as a precipitate, much as calcium deposits from tap water form when there is not enough water to keep them dissolved. A kidney stone can damage the lining of the urinary tract and cause bleeding and severe abdominal pain. Kidney stones are not unusual; it has been estimated that 1 million Americans have kidney stones and in 100,000 of the cases in any year the problem becomes serious enough to warrant hospitalization.

kilocalorie A unit of heat measure used in nutrition studies. It is the amount of heat required to raise the temperature of 1 kg. of water, slightly over 1 qt., by 1°C. Technically, the 1° temperature change must be from 15 to 16°C. Also called *kilogram calorie, large calorie*, or *Cal.* See *calorie; gram calorie*.

kilogram A measure of weight under the metric system of weights and measures. One kilogram is equal to 2.2 lb.

kinetic energy A term used to describe the energy involved in motion or action, as distinguished from *potential energy*, which is the ability to do work.

kosher A term that means foods selected and prepared in compliance with Jewish dietary laws. It is derived from the Hebrew word *kasher*, which means "good, fit, or proper." The dietary laws originally were public health measures intended to protect families from diseases and other adverse effects, such as malnutrition.

Kosher foods generally apply to three categories: inherently kosher foods, foods that are inherently not kosher, and foods that can become kosher if properly processed. Inherently kosher foods include the common plant food sources, such as fruits, vegetables, and cereals. Coffee and tea are also inherently kosher. Foods that are inherently not kosher include pork, birds of prey, and seafood that lacks fins and scales. Lobster, crabs, oysters, and eels are among those types of seafood. Foods that can become kosher if properly processed include most domestic meat and poultry products, excluding pork.

The processing of the meat from slaughtering of the animal to its appearance in a retail outlet is supervised by a rabbi or other qualified religious representative. The blood must be removed, using a procedure that involves soaking the carcass in cold water, salting it, allowing the blood to drain, then washing the meat again to remove the salt. The kosher custom of not serving meat and dairy products at the same meal reportedly originated as a symbolic reminder that if one takes both the meat and the milk from the animal at the same time, there may be none left to sustain future generations.

Krebiozen A substance promoted in the 1950s as a cancer "cure" derived from horse serum. The U.S. Food and Drug Administration banned the drug after studies showed the substance was *creatine*, a combination of three amino acids manufactured normally by the body and stored in muscle tissue and which has no effect on cancer.

Krebs cycle   The name given a series of steps that carbohydrates, amino acids, and fatty acids go through during the metabolic process, which eventually ends in the production of energy, carbon dioxide, and water. The cycle of reactions was discovered by a British biochemist, Hans Adolf Krebs. Also called *citric acid cycle*.

kwashiorkor   A disease condition that occurs in infants and young children who experience severe protein deficiency. Symptoms include fluid accumulation in the body tissues, retarded growth and development, pot belly, liver disorder, and marked changes in the color of the skin and hair. Kwashiorkor is prevalent in Third World countries where children may be weaned early, thereby interrupting their main supply of protein. *Kwashiorkor* is a West African word meaning "displaced child," the displaced child being the one who was weaned early to make room for another, younger brother or sister at the mother's breast.

lactase An enzyme needed in the small intestine to split molecules of lactose, or milk sugar, into the smaller sugar units of glucose and galactose, which can be absorbed through the intestinal wall. If the lactose molecules cannot be split, they remain in the digestive tract and accumulate water, resulting in symptoms of *lactose intolerance*. See this entry.

lactation The secretion of milk by the mammary glands. It is believed to result from the action of three hormones in the female body: estrogen, progesterone, and prolactin, which is also known as the lactogenic hormone. True lactation does not begin in the human mother until about 3 days after the baby has been delivered. During the few days immediately before and after birth, the breasts secrete a fluid called *colostrum*. See this entry.

lactose A type of sugar that occurs in the milk of mammals. It consists of 1 unit of glucose and 1 unit of galactose. Human milk is about 6 percent lactose; cow's milk contains a somewhat smaller amount. Lactose has the lowest level of sweetness of any of the common sugars and is tolerated by most people of northern European ancestry. However, many persons are unable to tolerate lactose in varying amounts. It is commonly used as an additive in baby foods, as a coating for foods, in the production of lactic acid, and in bakery products where it reacts with protein to form golden brown crusts on baked goods.

lactose intolerance A gastrointestinal disorder caused by the lack of an enzyme needed for digesting lactose, or milk sugar. People of northern European ancestry are generally not affected because they inherit a gene for producing the necessary enzyme, lactase. Black Americans, American Indians, and Orientals are the most commonly affected individuals. Symptoms include borborygmus or "gut rumblings," gas, cramps, diarrhea, nausea, and bloating. Some people are affected in a similar manner by a deficiency of other sugar-splitting enzymes.

large calorie An alternate term for *kilocalorie*, a measure of energy used by nutrition scientists, and equal to 1,000 small calories, or gram calories. See *calorie; gram calorie; kilocalorie.*

laryngeal cartilages A series of rings of cartilage that give shape to the larynx, or voice box, and that protect the vocal cords. The laryngeal cartilages also form the shape in the front of the neck, commonly known as the *Adam's apple.*

lateral hypothalamus An area of the brain that regulates the appetite. When the lateral hypothalamus tissues of experimental animals are stimulated by an electric current, the animals become increasingly hungry. But when the lateral hypothalamus is destroyed, the animals quit eating. See *appetite center.*

lead A metallic element that occurs naturally in soil, rocks, water, and air. Because of its presence in the environment, a significant amount accumulates in food and then in the blood and soft tissues of humans. The average amount of lead in a human adult has been calculated to be more than 1.5 parts per million, which is greater than the levels of some of the essential minerals present in the tissues. Lead is not essential to human life and can, in fact, cause serious damage to blood-forming, nervous, circulatory, urinary, gastrointestinal, and reproductive systems. Brain disease, palsy, anemia, and liver disorders are caused by lead in the body and large doses can be fatal.

lead in canned foods The residues of lead that enter the food supply through the use of older canning equipment in food processing plants. High levels of lead were of particular concern for users of canned milk in the 1970s, but the problem has diminished in recent years. See *tin.*

lecithin A substance found in all living plant and animal tissues and in the diet in such foods as eggs, corn, and soybeans. In the human body, lecithin is an important component of central nervous system tissues. Lecithin is also a common food additive, serving as an emulsifier for certain bakery products, chocolate confections, and frozen desserts, as an antioxidant in cereals and bakery products, and as a defoaming agent in sugar beet processing.

left-handed sugar A common name given to sugar molecules that are almost identical to ordinary sugars, such as glucose and fructose, except that they are mirror images. Naturally occurring sugars are right handed, which is why glucose is also known as dextrose. Left-handed sugar is a man-made carbohydrate that manufacturers claim is as sweet as table sugar, but without the calories.

leiomyoma A type of noncancerous tumor that may develop in the lower half of the esophagus, resulting in discomfort in eating and swallowing foods. A leiomyoma usually causes more difficulty when eating solid foods than in swallowing liquids. It can be removed by surgery, although radiation is sometimes an option.

leucine   An essential amino acid that occurs in most food proteins. It is found in various tissues of the human body and is essential for normal growth. Eggs, casein, soybeans, and wheat gluten are rich sources of leucine.

leukocytes   A word for white blood cells which combines two Greek words: *leukos*, meaning "white," and *kytos*, or "cell." See *blood cells; white blood cells*.

leukoplakia   A white plaque that may form in the membranes lining the mouth, often in association with heavy use of alcoholic beverages and tobacco. The plaques frequently subside when drinking and smoking are curtailed and the mouth is properly cared for, including brushing the teeth regularly. If the plaques are not treated early they may develop into cancers.

levulose   See *fructose*.

lichen planus   A disease of the mucous membrane lining the mouth. It often appears as a pattern of white lacy lesions on the tongue, palate, and other inner surfaces of the mouth. It is caused by a microorganism complex that is part fungi and part algae. The same microorganism may cause problems in other body areas, where there is hair or nail surface. The disease may persist for weeks or months, then suddenly disappear, with or without treatment. It sometimes responds to treatments of vitamin A.

licorice   An herb that originated in the Mediterranean region but has spread to wet, wild areas of all continents. Licorice roots, powders, and extracts are used as flavoring additives for soft drinks, ice creams, chewing gums, candies, and bakery products. Artificial maple and root beer flavors may depend on a touch of licorice extract. Although licorice can cause increased blood pressure and other effects in some people, it has been used as a medicinal herb since ancient times and has been found with other folk remedies in the tombs of the Pharaohs.

light diet   The name used for any diet of simple, mixed food items suitable for a bed patient or one who is recovering from a serious illness or injury and gets little exercise.

lignin   A type of plant fiber that is usually a part of the cell wall structure of fruits and vegetables, particularly in older or mature plant food sources. Cell walls of young plants are generally thin and composed mainly of cellulose. Lignin gradually replaces the cellulose with thick, tough fibers that resist softening by cooking and are difficult to chew.

limiting amino acid An essential amino acid that is not present in sufficient quantity in a food protein to make possible full utilization of the protein. Unless a protein supplies all eight essential amino acids in the right proportions needed by the body, the amino acid that is disproportionately lowest will limit the other seven amino acids by an equivalent amount. This deficiency of the limiting amino acid can be overcome by using *complementary proteins*. See this entry.

lingual tonsils The name of a mass of tonsil tissue at the root of the tongue. The tonsils may appear as anywhere from a few dozen to as many as 100 elevations on the rear one-third of the tongue. They are composed of lymphatic tissue and serve the purpose of screening microorganisms that may enter the mouth.

linoleic acid An unsaturated fatty acid essential for humans and animals. It occurs naturally in vegetable oils, primarily corn, cottonseed, linseed, soy, and wheat-germ oils. A deficiency of linoleic acid in animal experiments results in a cessation of growth, kidney damage, skin disorders, and loss of reproductive ability.

linolenic acid An unsaturated fatty acid obtained from linseed oil. It is also synthesized in the human body from linoleic acid. In animal experiments, researchers have discovered that health effects caused by a deficiency of linoleic acid, such as skin and kidney disorders, could be corrected by adding it to their diets.

lipase The name of any of a group of enzymes produced by the body for the purpose of breaking down fats. Specific lipases are secreted by the stomach, liver, pancreas, and intestinal tract. The general function of lipases is to break down triglyceride molecules into fatty acid and glycerol molecules.

lipid A term applied to any substance that can be dissolved in a fat solvent, such as ether or alcohol, but cannot be dissolved in water. This category includes fatty acids, neutral fats, waxes, glycerides, steroids, such as sex hormones, and fat-soluble vitamins, particularly vitamin D. The term is derived from the Greek word *lipos*, meaning "fat."

lipoic acid A coenzyme found in liver and yeast that plays a role in the digestion of carbohydrates. It has been identified by some nutritionists as a vitamin but others contend it is not, and no human requirement for the substance has been established.

liquid vitamins Vitamin supplements prepared in liquid form, mainly for children and for adults who have difficulty swallowing or chewing tablets. Liquid vitamins may be supplied with a calibrated dropper so that precise amounts of the preparation can be measured. Because the normal human body adjusts itself to usual intakes of vitamin supplements by storing or excreting any excesses, liquid vitamins are not generally promoted to the general public.

liter A liquid measure used in the metric system of weights and measures. It is roughly equivalent to 1 qt.

lithium A nonessential mineral found in trace amounts in the human body. It is the lightest metallic element and also the lightest of all chemical elements that is a solid at room temperature.

liver A large, dark-reddish gland located in the upper right part of the abdomen; sometimes it can be felt just below the bottom edge of the chest cage of ribs. It is the largest gland in the body, measuring about 10 in. in width and weighing 3 lb.

It contains millions of specialized cells that are involved in most of the metabolic processes of the body. The liver receives blood from two major vessels. One is the *hepatic artery*, which delivers freshly oxygenated blood almost directly from the heart. The other is the *portal vein*, which carries the assorted nutrients and nonnutrients absorbed from the intestinal tract. Among the nutrients received are carbohydrate molecules that may need further processing to become glucose units, amino acids that must be sorted into those that can be used directly and those that must be broken down into other molecules for energy or for spare parts for proteins, and fatty acids, which are treated similarly.

Because the liver also has the task of cleaning out toxic substances in the diet, it possesses enzymes that neutralize nonnutrients. Caffeine molecules from coffee, for example, are broken down into less-toxic substances that can be excreted quickly. Too much of a toxic chemical, however, can overload the liver's enzyme systems and be the cause of liver degeneration. One example is the excessive use of alcohol for a long period of time; the liver enzymes can cope with a small-to-moderate amount of alcohol, but too much of the chemical causes the disease known as *cirrhosis*. Other functions of the liver include blood storage and bile production. The liver contains reservoirs that can hold as much as 6 pt. of blood for emergency use. Bile is routed back to the intestines to help break down fatty foods.

low-calorie diet Any diet that provides 1,200 calories or less per day. Such diets are hard to plan and maintain because of the difficulty people have finding interesting foods that contain few calories but also provide all the essential nutrients, including vitamins and minerals. Because most people burn more than 1,200 calories per day through basal metabolic activities, like maintaining a normal body temperature, a 1,200-calorie diet requires a doctor's supervision.

low-cholesterol diet A diet for people who have a high level of cholesterol in their blood and who may be likely candidates for coronary heart disease. The diet emphasizes an increase in polyunsaturated fats and a decrease in saturated fats in foods. Among restricted foods are commercial hot chocolate, cereals with coconut, butter rolls, cheese bread, doughnuts, cornbread, muffins, biscuits, French toast, ice cream, commercial pastries, pies, and puddings, unless they are made only with polyunsaturated vegetable oils.

low-fat diet A diet that contains a minimum amount of fat. One type of fat diet designed for persons afflicted with gall bladder disorders restricts total fat intake to 45 g. per day without considering specific kinds of fatty acids. Excluded are avocados, bacon, fried or grilled meats, cured or canned meats, duck, goose, fried eggs, all canned or commercial soups, all milks except skim milk and buttermilk, and all smoked fish or fish canned in oil. A low-fat diet may also exclude strong-flavored vegetables and high-fiber foods.

lower-fiber diet A diet designed mainly for people about to undergo intestinal surgery or colon exploration by colonoscopy. It eliminates all whole-grain breads or rolls; all barley, bran, or whole-grain cereals; all bakery products containing fruits, nuts, skins, or seeds; all fried foods, including fried eggs; all spiced or pickled meats; and all raw fruits, except bananas.

low-potassium diet A diet that may be required for patients with adrenal insufficiency disorders, such as Addison's disease, in which potassium accumulates to high levels in the body while sodium is excreted at an abnormally rapid rate. This diet restricts the use of such items as meat, fish, poultry, milk and milk products, coffee, bran and whole-wheat products, molasses, canned soups containing dried beans, peas, or lentils, baked beans, lima beans, broccoli, fresh carrots, kale, white or sweet potatoes, tomatoes, spinach, and a variety of fruits from apricots and avocados to prunes and fresh pears.

low-protein diet A diet designed for persons who must restrict their intake of protein for various reasons, such as abnormal protein metabolism caused by severe liver disease or kidney failure. Low-protein diets are based on individual body weights and may restrict protein intake to 40 g. per day, with the protein foods distributed over several meals. Caloric intake meanwhile is very high in order to maintain a protein-sparing effect, which makes the body utilize a lot of carbohydrates and fats so that protein metabolism will be reduced.

low-residue diet A diet that results in the least possible amount of feces. Such a diet usually consists of gelatins, broths, simple sugars like sucrose and glucose, boiled eggs, meats, liver, cottage cheese, and rice.

low-salt diet   A moderate form of a low-sodium diet, in which the person eliminates the use of table salt on his food and/or restricts his use of highly salted or salt-preserved foods. The average North American uses between 4,000 and 6,000 mg. of sodium daily, mainly in the form of salted foods. See *low-sodium diet*.

low-sodium diet   A diet that severely restricts the use of sodium in any form, but particularly sodium chloride, because of its tendency to aggravate high blood pressure, congestive heart failure, and kidney and liver diseases marked by fluid accumulation. A severely restricted low-sodium diet may limit total sodium intake per day to 250 mg., little more than 1/10 the amount in 1 tsp. of table salt. Two slices of regular bread, ½ cup of regular cottage cheese, a bowl of dry cereal, or a glass of chocolate milk would use up the day's ration of sodium in food; each item would contain about 250 mg. of the mineral.

lumpy jaw   The common name for a type of fungal disease that invades the mouth and causes the formation of lumps in the soft tissues. The lumps contain pus and usually require antibiotic treatments or surgery, or both.

lymph   A transparent, yellowish fluid that is about 95 percent water and is found within the vessels of the body's lymphatic system. It accumulates in the lymphatic vessels from tissues in all parts of the body and is returned to the blood circulatory system, where it originated. Lymph contains plasma proteins and other chemicals normally dissolved in the blood plasma, plus lymphocytes. It represents the fluid portion of the blood that is allowed to seep through the capillary walls and into the body tissues as the blood circulates throughout the body; it returns via the lymphatic vessels that empty into the large veins at the base of the neck.

lysine   One of the essential amino acids. Most protein food sources contain lysine, but it is more abundant in the muscle meats of fish, fowl, beef, pork, and lamb. Among the better plant sources are soybeans, spinach, and beet greens.

m

macroelement A mineral required by adult humans in amounts greater than 100 mg. (about 1/300 of 1 oz.) per day. Calcium, phosphorus, magnesium, and sodium are macroelements.

macroglossia A deformity of the tongue in which it becomes so large that it interferes with the normal functions of the mouth, such as speaking and eating. The overgrown tongue can be reshaped by a surgeon to fit the mouth without obstructing normal mouth activities.

magnesium One of the minerals required by the human body in relatively significant amounts. Even though the average human can function normally on a total of less than 1 oz. of magnesium, that amount is still thousands to hundreds of thousands of times larger than some of the microelements or trace minerals needed to support a single function of an enzyme or vitamin.

Magnesium is used mainly in the human body in compounds that form bone structures; about 70 percent of the magnesium is combined with calcium and phosphorus in the skeleton. The rest of the body's magnesium supply enters into various enzyme functions, such as those involved in the burning of sugar calories at the level of individual tissue cells.

A deficiency of magnesium is characterized by disorders of the muscular and nervous systems, with symptoms that include muscle spasms and tremors and, in severe cases, convulsions. Although deficiencies in humans are rare in people with proper health habits, they can develop in alcoholics and others whose eating habits fail to include adequate amounts of legumes, such as beans and peas, whole-grain cereals, green leafy vegetables, and nuts. Cocoa and chocolate also are good sources of magnesium. Certain diseases, such as kidney disorders and malabsorption syndromes, may also affect normal daily intake of magnesium.

The recommended daily allowance (RDA) of magnesium is between 300 and 350 mg. Three ounces of cocoa, probably the richest source, should provide about 360 mg. of magnesium; an equivalent amount of almonds or cashews would contribute around 250 mg. Overdoses of magnesium can cause diarrhea, but excess amounts are generally not harmful to a healthy human.

magnesium carbonate   A white powder present in dolomite and used as an additive in a variety of processed foods, such as sour cream and ice cream, chocolate manufacture, and canned vegetables. Its alkaline properties have been utilized in antacid remedies.

magnesium oxide   A common dietary form of magnesium, which, like magnesium carbonate, is used in processed foods, such as dairy products, chocolate, and canned vegetables. It may also be used in certain laxative and antacid preparations.

magnesium sulfate   Small, colorless crystals with a bitter taste that may be used in laxatives, poultices, and anticonvulsant medications. It is also used in hot water as a soak for sore and strained muscles. In food processing, magnesium sulfate may be used in the manufacture of beer. Also called *Epsom salts*.

malabsorption   The failure or inability of nutrients to pass through the walls of the small intestine and into the bloodstream for further metabolism. There are two dozen specific causes of malabsorption, including inadequate digestion of food items by gastric juices, celiac disease, radiation injury to the lining of the intestine, parasitic diseases, hormonal disorders, obstruction of the lymphatic vessels draining nutrients from the intestinal tract, and enzyme deficiencies. Signs and symptoms of malabsorption vary with the specific disorder, but may include cramps, diarrhea, weakness and lack of endurance, poor appetite and weight loss, bone pain, sore tongue, skin eruptions, and pot belly. See *inborn errors of metabolism; glucose-galactose malabsorption; celiac-sprue; idiopathic steatorrhea*.

malabsorption syndrome   A medical term for a group of disorders characterized by abnormal absorption of nutrients from the intestine and their loss by excretion, resulting in a variety of nutrient deficiency symptoms. See *malabsorption*.

malic acid   An acid found in the juices of fruits and other plant materials and a by-product of carbohydrate metabolism in the human body. It is also a food additive used in wines, jellies, jams, and other products that require an acidic, fruity flavor. Apples are a common natural source of malic acid.

malnutrition   A condition of poor nourishment caused by an improper diet or a bodily defect that prevents it from using foods properly. Malnutrition may be the result of too much food as well as a lack of food, but poverty and lack of knowledge of nutrition are important factors. Weight-loss diets, misguided vegetarianism, and cultural food taboos may be causes of malnutrition in populations that have easy access to proper nutrients. In some parts of the world, for example, people have cows but do not consume the meat or milk for religious or other reasons. Similarly, other people raise chickens but do not eat eggs for religious or cultural reasons.

maltase   A sugar-splitting enzyme that occurs in the intestinal tract and has the job of splitting each maltose molecule into two glucose molecules.

maltose   A form of sugar commonly found in sprouting grains. It is also produced during the digestion of starch. A maltose molecule consists of two glucose units, and further digestion of maltose yields glucose, the basic unit of carbohydrates. Maltose is an easily digestible type of sugar and is often used in infant formulas.

manganese   A mineral that occurs in very small amounts in the human body (approximately 1 part per 5-million), mainly in the bones, liver, and pituitary gland. Manganese serves as a cofactor of vitamin K in the synthesis of blood-clotting factors and also as a cofactor in many enzyme functions related to the metabolism of carbohydrates, fats, and proteins. In protein metabolism, it plays a role in the production of urea from nitrogen waste products. Food sources are green vegetables, legumes, nuts, and cereals.

manipulation   A technique for restoring function to an arm or leg by moving it through at least a part of the range of motion permitted by the joint.

mannitol   A sugar-alcohol substance that occurs widely in nature. Fungi are usually rich sources of mannitol. The mannitol used in food processing usually comes from seaweed. It is used mainly in candy and chewing gum and as a sweet-tasting, odorless dusting on other food products. Mannitol is employed as a sweetener in diet beverages and similar products as an alternative to sugar. Although it is technically a sugar, it is not as easily fermented as common sugars and therefore is less likely to be a cause of dental decay.

mannose   A simple sugar derived from mannitol with properties similar to those of glucose. Although it is named for the manna tree, which is native to the Mediterranean region, the mannose used in food processing is obtained from the vegetable ivory nut, the fruit of a South American palm tree.

marasmus   A form of childhood malnutrition, similar to kwashiorkor, that occurs primarily in the first year of life. Symptoms include growth retardation and a wasting of muscles and subcutaneous fat. Marasmus differs from kwashiorkor in that the cause of malnutrition is one of calorie deficiency, in addition to protein deficiency. See *kwashiorkor*.

marginal deficiency   A deficiency of one or more minerals or other nutrients in the diet that is not serious enough to be a major health risk but may prevent a person from enjoying optimum health. One example of a marginal deficiency is an inadequate intake of zinc that results in a slower rate of healing of a cut in the skin, but which is not so inadequate as to produce obvious deficiency symptoms.

masseter   One of the groups of muscles that helps move the lower jaw when chewing food. It consists of a powerful set of muscle fibers attached at one end to the part of the upper jaw just below the eye, on either side of the head, and to the back of the lower jaw at the other end.

mastication   A technical term for the act of chewing food. The term is derived from an ancient Greek word meaning "to gnash the teeth."

MDR   See *minimum daily requirement*.

meat tenderizers   Substances added to meats to break down the tough fibers. A common meat tenderizer is *papain*, an enzyme extracted from the papaya fruit. The meat tenderizer is applied to the meat before cooking because heat deactivates the enzyme. Other meat tenderizers include *ficin*, an enzyme obtained from certain fig trees, and *bromelin*, which is obtained from raw pineapple juice. Bromelin is such a powerful enzyme that people who handle cut raw pineapple must wear gloves to protect their hands; like papain, the pineapple enzyme is deactivated by heat.

Medicaid   The common name for a 1965 U.S. Social Security law that authorizes the federal government to provide matching funds to states to help finance health care for people who are on welfare or are otherwise unable to pay for medical services. The services and money available for Medicaid coverage are determined by the individual state's plan, which varies from state to state.

Medicare   A two-part U.S. Social Security program designed to provide a form of health insurance for older persons. One part pays for basic costs of hospitalization and related services, such as home health care after release from a hospital. The second part is a voluntary health insurance program, financed with the help of contributions from Social Security recipients, that pays for physician services and certain health care costs not covered by the first part.

medium-chain triglyceride   A dietary form of fat called MCT that is manufactured for persons unable to absorb certain fatty acids. See *idiopathic steatorrhea*.

megadose vitamins Daily vitamin doses that are many times the amount of the RDAs. Megadoses of vitamins, sometimes as much as 25 to 50 times the RDA, have been used experimentally in treating certain disorders; however, the effects have varied with different individuals and the subject remains controversial.

megavitamin therapy The use of megadoses of vitamins to treat certain health problems. Because vitamins do have biological effects, they are sometimes used by physicians as drugs rather than for simply preventing deficiency diseases. Niacin, for example, may be prescribed in megadose levels to lower the cholesterol level in a patient with heart disease. Megavitamin therapy is conducted under the supervision of a physician who is able to monitor the precise effects and who is also aware of the biochemistry of the vitamin and how it may interact with other substances in the body when administered in greater than RDA amounts.

menstruation The normal periodic discharge of blood from the vagina due to the sloughing-off of blood-rich cells that line the uterus during the child-bearing years of a woman's life. The event occurs on the average of once every 28 days, although the cycle for some women may occur at intervals of less than or more than 28 days and may vary for individual women. Menstruation usually begins after age 11 and continues, except for pregnancies, until menopause, which may begin in the forties. Menstruation results in a loss of from 15 to 30 mg. of iron, which should be accounted for in the diet in addition to the normal daily loss of 1 mg. daily for both men and women.

mercury A nonessential and potentially toxic mineral that enters the body through the food supply. The average human adult body contains about 1 part per 5-million of mercury. Pure metallic mercury is not poisonous because it is not absorbed by the body. However, mercury combines easily with other substances, such as the chloride ion, to form salts that are fatal in amounts as small as 1 g. (about 1/30 of 1 oz.). Mercury is used in diuretics and other medications, such as calomel, and enters the food supply through fish that live in contaminated waters and seed grains treated with mercury pesticides.

metabolism The physical and chemical activities and reactions that occur among the atoms, molecules, and ions in the body in connection with the processes associated with the digestion and assimilation of food. Metabolism occurs in two phases, called *anabolism* and *catabolism*. Anabolism is the phase concerned with the use of nutrients for building and repairing body tissues. Catabolism is the tearing down of molecules into simpler substances and in the release of energy stored in food molecules. The two phases usually work in harmony as many nutrients, such as amino acids, must be broken down into simpler units so they can be reorganized as new body proteins.

metenoic acid A substance promoted as vitamin U and reported to provide relief for ulcers. However, claims to its status as a vitamin have been challenged by authorities. Metenoic acid has been identified as a substance extracted from cabbage juice and is probably derived from a form of the amino acid methionine.

methionine An essential amino acid important in the normal growth of infants. It is also required in adults to maintain nitrogen equilibrium. Methionine is also used in special dietary supplements used for therapeutic purposes. Although the body is unable to synthesize methionine, it can be manufactured by food processors. It occurs naturally in all the usual protein foods but some, like eggs, are better sources than others. Rice is one of the better plant food sources of methionine. Methionine is utilized by the body in the manufacture of insulin molecules and in the formation of keratin, the horny substance of hair and nails.

methylcellulose A substance made from cellulose that is used as a bulk laxative and as a weight-control product. Methylcellulose absorbs water and swells to several times its original size in the digestive tract. It is also used as a thickening agent in certain food products.

microelement A term sometimes used to identify nutrients which humans require each day in amounts that are less than 100 mg. (about 1/300 of 1 oz.) Actually, most minerals and vitamins are required in microelement amounts.

microgram A weight measure in the metric system that is 1/1,000,000 of 1 g. or approximately 1/30,000,000 of 1 oz. A few microelements, such as manganese and molybdenum and vitamins A and D, are measured in micrograms of daily intake. Abbreviated μg.

micronutrients The inorganic elements, or minerals, needed by the body in extremely small amounts. Also called *trace elements.* See *microelements.*

microwave An electromagnetic radiation, similar to that used in radar and radio or TV broadcasting but with wavelengths of between 1 mm. and 30 cm. Microwaves are used in cooking by agitating the water molecules in foods and causing an increase in temperature simultaneously throughout the food item. Heating is rapid and microwave cooking is generally about 10 times as fast as conventional baking or other cooking methods. Microwave heating is also used in commercial food processing to thaw meats and other foods that have been frozen for storage purposes.

migraine A type of headache that is usually severe and often affects only one side of the head. It is sometimes accompanied by nausea and vomiting.

Symptoms vary among different individuals and may occur during the menstrual period in women. Some individuals experience light flashes or flickering or a partial loss of vision at the start of a migraine attack. Attacks are associated with constriction and dilation of the cerebral arteries and they seem to be aggravated by emotional upsets.

milk A fluid form of nutrition produced in the mammary glands of many species of mammals for the primary purpose of nursing their offspring. In North America, most milk produced for commercial purposes comes from cows, although small amounts may come from goats. Cow's milk averages about 87 percent water, 5 percent lactose (milk sugar), 4 percent butterfat, 3 percent protein, and less than 1 percent minerals; exact amounts vary somewhat, with milk from Guernsey and Jersey cows containing more butterfat than milk from Holstein cows. Human milk contains more lactose, vitamin E, and food energy than cow's milk.

milk allergy A severe sensitivity to milk, particularly cow's milk, because of intolerance to lactose, or milk sugar, or to a protein in milk. People whose ancestors were from northern Europe usually inherit an enzyme that allows them to digest milk sugar without difficulty, but many others, including most blacks, Orientals, and American Indians, lack the enzyme and as a result experience diarrhea, nausea, cramps, or other effects when the milk sugar ferments in their digestive tracts. Other people allergic to milk protein experience diarrhea, vomiting, and bloody feces when they drink milk. Milk-allergy patients need to find substitutes, such as soy milk, to obtain the nutrients others get from cow's milk.

milk sugar A common name for lactose, one of a very few types of carbohydrates produced by animals. See *lactose*.

milligram A unit of weight in the metric system that is 1/1,000 of 1 g. or about 1/30,000 of 1 oz.

mineralocorticoid A term used to identify any of the hormones of the adrenal cortex that affect electrolytes, such as sodium, potassium, and chloride. A mineralocorticoid deficiency can result in such effects as an excessive loss of sodium and water in the urine and retention of potassium in the extracellular fluids rather than within the cells. The most important mineralocorticoid is aldosterone.

mineral oil A mixture of liquid hydrocarbons obtained from petroleum. Light mineral oil is used as a vehicle for certain medications and sometimes as a laxative and in skin-cleansing preparations. Heavy mineral oil may also be used in certain laxative formulations. Mineral oil is usually not recommended for internal use unless necessary because it interferes with the absorption of fat-soluble vitamins.

mineral A term usually applied to any solid inorganic chemical element, although the term is often broadened to include certain inorganic electrolytes or substances that are generally not solid at room temperature, such as chlorine. There are at least 20 different minerals found in the human body and more than a dozen of them are believed to be essential for normal health.

mineral salts Salts formed by the combination of minerals with other elements, such as the combination of sodium and chlorine in sodium chloride, or table salt, or potassium and iodine in potassium iodide, the substance added to table salt to make it iodized salt.

mineral supplements Tablets, capsules, or other preparations sold with or without a prescription that contain minerals essential for normal health. Mineral supplements are often sold in combination with vitamin supplements and the number and amounts of minerals may vary, although the label on the container lists the minerals and the dosages in RDA percentages. Mineral supplements are a convenient means of ensuring that an individual obtains adequate levels of essential nutrients when they may not be available from the foods chosen by the person for his meals.

mineral water Water that contains a high concentration of dissolved minerals in it. The specific minerals and amounts vary widely among the commercial mineral waters, some of which are ordinary drinking water to which minerals have been added. Some mineral waters contain dissolved substances that are not necessarily beneficial, including arsenic, cadmium, lead, and sodium. Most North American mineral waters contain the same elements as the well-promoted European mineral waters.

minimum daily requirements The daily human requirements established by the U.S. Food and Drug Administration as the amounts of nutrients, such as vitamins and minerals, needed to prevent a deficiency plus amounts that provide a small margin of safety. Abbreviated *MDR*. See *recommended dietary allowances*.

modified food starches Natural plant starches that are converted by food processors to make them suitable for packaged foods, such as cake flours. Some flours for baking may contain as much as 15 percent modified starch as a substitute for sugar or shortening. Modified starches are also used as thickeners and stabilizers for fillings, toppings, gravies, stews, and sauces. They are used in some baby foods, presumably because they are easier for children to digest than natural starches. Use of these starches has been a source of controversy because of the chemicals used to modify them.

molds A group of microscopic fungi that consist of branched threads of cells shaped like tiny tubes united end to end. Because molds grow best in an acidic environment, they are attracted to fruit. Molds spread in a vinelike manner and reproduce by showering the area with spores. Mold effects are usually obvious because of the cottony appearance of their presence on fruits and the loss of firm texture and sweet flavor. Some molds, such as aflatoxins, produce a poisonous substance that can cause cancer.

molybdenum A mineral used in the human body as a cofactor of several enzymes, including one that forms uric acid. It is present in the body at a level of about 1 part per 10-million. Molybdenum is believed to be involved in the metabolism of iron. It is an antimetabolite of copper, substituting for and interfering with copper functions in body tissues. Sulfur in foods increases the rate of excretion of molybdenum, apparently by blocking the kidney's normal action of retaining the mineral. Organ meats, milk, leafy vegetables, cereals, and legumes are food sources of molybdenum. However, an increased intake of molybdenum produces gout symptoms by increasing uric acid levels in the blood.

monoamine oxidase inhibitors Drugs, sometimes called "psychic energizers," that are used in the treatment of psychological depression and certain other disorders. People who are prescribed these drugs must avoid certain foods that interact with them, such as aged cheeses and Chianti wines, because they contain a substance known as *tyramine*. Tyramine is a metabolic by-product of the amino acid tyrosine and is a chemical cousin of several adrenal gland hormones. When monoamine oxidase, an enzyme, is inhibited by the drug, which normally metabolizes tyramine, the tyramine accumulates in the body, causing dangerously high levels of blood pressure, headaches, and other adverse effects.

monobasic ammonium phosphate An odorless white powder used in baking powder with sodium bicarbonate. Ammonium phosphates are also used in purifying sugar, culturing yeast, baking bread, and in beer manufacture.

monosaccharide A technical term for a simple sugar that cannot be broken down into simpler units. Glucose, or dextrose, is an example of a monosaccharide. When two monosaccharides are combined in a bigger sugar molecule, it becomes a disaccharide.

monosodium glutamate A white powder that is a chemical compound of sodium and the amino acid, glutamic acid. It occurs naturally in many plants, particularly seaweed, and is the reason why seaweed was used for centuries as a flavoring ingredient. Today, it is manufactured from wheat gluten, as a by-product of beet sugar, and from casein, as well as from seaweed and soybeans. Alone, monosodium glutamate has a salty taste, but when added in small amounts to gravies, sauces, meats, bouillons, and protein-rich foods it improves the flavor. In larger amounts, it can have adverse health effects, such as the *Chinese restaurant syndrome*. See this entry. Abbreviated MSG.

mouth A word that means an opening and is generally used to identify the opening into the digestive tract. The primary function of the human mouth is one of chewing food—with the teeth, taste buds, saliva glands, and tongue participating in the activity. The mouth also helps to shape the sound of the voice and is an auxiliary source of air for breathing when the nasal passages are blocked. Although the teeth are commonly associated with mastication, the tongue also plays an important role, as it is used to move the food in the mouth into the appropriate areas of teeth for tearing and grinding. It also helps pulverize the food by pushing it against the hard palate at the roof of the mouth.

mouth-feel The sensations of texture, shape, temperature, and other factors that help a person judge the type and quality of food in the mouth without actually seeing it. Companies that manufacture food products are particularly interested in creating foods that have an attractive mouth-feel. Most people develop mouth-feel associations for certain foods at an early age and expect that a milk shake, cheeseburger, or breakfast cereal—even if synthesized from food additives, modified starch, or other substances—will have the mouth-feel of the real thing.

MSG See *monosodium glutamate; Chinese restaurant syndrome.*

mucocele A cyst that can develop on the inner surface of the membranes of the lips or cheeks. The cyst can be very soft or quite hard and generally it keeps growing until it is removed by surgery.

multivitamin supplements Any vitamin supplement preparation that contains two or more vitamins.

muscular rheumatism See *myalgia.*

muscle-building foods Foods that are good sources of essential amino acids, which are needed as building blocks for muscle proteins. However, simply eating foods rich in amino acids will not build muscle tissue unless the muscles are exercised regularly and vigorously. Otherwise, the amino acids are simply converted into fuel to provide body heat and maintain basic metabolic functions. Once muscles are developed, carbohydrates become an important source of energy for efficient muscle power.

mutagenic Anything capable of causing a mutation, or alteration, in hereditary traits. A true mutation involves the creation of a new gene, or bit of hereditary material, that can be transmitted to children and grandchildren. Most human mutations arise spontaneously, without a known cause. Because certain chemicals can produce mutations, some food additives are now tested for several generations of animals to determine whether they might be possible causes of human mutations.

myalgia A medical term for tenderness or pain in the muscle tissue. Also called *muscular rheumatism*.

myelin A fatty substance that forms a protective sheath around certain nerve fibers, mainly the nerves that originate in the brain and spinal cord. Myelin allows nerve impulses to travel more rapidly and efficiently. In a number of nervous system diseases, the cause is traced to a loss of myelin from the nerves.

myocardial infarction The medical term for a heart attack. It means that a part of the heart muscle has been killed or severely damaged by an interruption of blood carrying oxygen to the muscle tissue. An interruption of the supply of fresh blood to tissue cells in any part of the body for more than a moment can result in the death of the cells, which in effect are suffocated. An obstruction of a blood vessel by a clot or a break or rupture in a blood vessel wall can result in an infarction.

myoglobin A substance similar to the hemoglobin of red blood cells that is present in muscle tissue. Myoglobin allows the muscle to store oxygen and it contributes to the reddish color of muscle tissue. Meats are sometimes classified as either red muscle or white muscle, the red muscle representing tissues that are rich in myoglobin.

n

natural vitamin supplements Vitamin tablets or capsules containing vitamins obtained from fish oils, yeast, dried liver, or bone marrow. There is no evidence that the vitamins obtained directly from plants and animals are physiologically different or superior to synthetic vitamins containing the same amounts of the same substances. However, the "natural" vitamins may be more expensive because of the difficulty of extracting vitamin C from rose hips, for example, as compared to using ascorbic acid, which is the same substance and produces the same effects.

nephritic diet A diet for persons afflicted with kidney inflammation. It restricts nitrogen-rich foods, such as proteins, and prohibits spicy foods, alcoholic beverages, and the use of condiments in general. In some cases of severe kidney disease, nitrogen foods are limited to those providing the essential amino acids.

neurotransmitter A chemical messenger that carries a nerve impulse from one nerve fiber to another. Nerves are generally separated along nervous system pathways by a gap called a *synapse*. Unless a neurotransmitter is available to help the nerve impulse across the gap, it may travel no farther. Neurotransmitters include substances with names like *dopamine, norepinephrine, acetylcholine, glutamate, serotonin,* and *GABA* (gamma-aminobutyric acid). See these entries.

niacin An important water-soluble vitamin of the B-complex found in a wide variety of plant and animal food sources, ranging from fish, poultry, and lean meats, to yeast, bran, and peanuts. A deficiency of niacin causes a disease known for hundreds of years as *pellagra*, a term derived from an Italian word for "rough skin." One of the symptoms of pellagra is a rough, red skin. Pellagra also causes mental health and digestive tract problems. It can also be fatal. In the United States alone, as many as 10,000 deaths annually were attributed to pellagra before doctors realized that the disease could be cured with niacin.

Pellagra occurred in families that depended on corn as a regular item in their meals. In the rural South of the United States, a bushel of corn would feed almost two dozen people who could not afford protein-rich foods. The corn meal diet was often supplemented with molasses, ham fat, and lard, none of which was a source of niacin. Pellagra, which acquired its name in Italy, caused similar problems in European countries that had been growing corn as a cereal staple since it was introduced shortly after the discovery of the New World. Corn was the obvious culprit as far as most physicians were concerned, but they insisted that the real cause of the disease was something that contaminated the corn, such as a bacteria or mold. (Until recent years, physicians received no training in nutrition and little was known about vitamin deficiency diseases.)

Ironically, niacin, which is also known as nicotinic acid, had been synthesized by a nineteenth-century German chemist from nicotine, the poisonous alkaloid in tobacco. But nobody recognized at the time that nicotinic acid was the same substance needed to prevent pellagra. Also overlooked at the time was the fact that many of the families that subsisted mainly on corn escaped the effects of pellagra because they drank a lot of fresh, black coffee; the coffee beans contained small amounts of niacin. Still another part of the niacin picture was a tendency of some dogs to develop a disease called *black tongue*, which could be cured by giving the dogs nicotinic acid. Black tongue, it was discovered some time later, is simply a canine version of pellagra.

Niacin had been isolated and identified in extracts of yeast and rice bran in England and Japan in 1912, but overlooked at the time because scientists were searching for the cause of beriberi. It was not until the 1930s that other researchers in Germany and the United States began to put together the varied pieces of the puzzle. They realized that the substance in yeast, rice bran, and coffee beans was the element missing from foods eaten by people and dogs that resulted in pellagra symptoms, and that nicotinic acid, niacinamide, and niacin were different names for the same missing element. Within 10 years, pellagra became a rare disease. The cause and cure were so simple they had been overlooked by everybody.

The primary function of niacin in the body is to serve as a coenzyme, mainly in oxidation reactions in the tissue cells. Without niacin, all cells of the body can suffer. Among the best sources of niacin are peanut butter, beef and calves' liver, canned tuna and salmon, whole wheat, and meats. The body can also manufacture niacin from tryptophan in the diet. The name of the vitamin, niacin, was adopted at the request of the American Medical Association, which objected to the use of the term, nicotinic acid, because it revealed the relationship between the vitamin and nicotine. Also called *nicotinic acid; vitamin B-5*. See *niacin equivalent; niacinamide; pellagra*.

niacinamide A form of niacin that is often used in vitamin supplements and antipellagra preparations because it does not cause dilation of the arteries, which is an effect of pure niacin. Niacinamide and niacin are interconvertible, that is, one can be converted into the other form by the body's chemical mechanisms.

niacin equivalent   A term used by nutrition experts to express a relationship between niacin, a B vitamin, and the amino acid, tryptophan, which can be converted by the human body to niacin. The body can produce 1 mg. of niacin from 60 mg. of tryptophan. Therefore, one niacin equivalent could be either 1 mg. of niacin or 60 mg. of tryptophan.

nickel   A mineral believed to be involved in the structure and function of liver tissues, particularly the functions related to fat metabolism. Nickel appears to be released from body stores during periods of physical stress, such as high fever, heart attack, stroke, or severe burns.

nicotinamide   An alternative term for *niacinamide*. See this entry.

nicotine   A potentially lethal poison obtained as a pungent, oily liquid from tobacco plants. A fatal dose of pure nicotine is about 40 mg., the amount in a single drop of the substance and the amount contained in two cigarettes. However, smoking tobacco burns most of the nicotine and not enough is absorbed by the body to cause death. Nicotine in tobacco can cause digestive upsets, increased blood pressure, and central nervous system changes. It is used in a large number of insect poisons.

nicotinic acid   The original name of niacin. Nicotinic acid was discovered in 1867 by German chemists when they added oxygen to the nicotine extracted from tobacco leaves. Nearly 70 years later it was found that nicotinic acid was identical to niacin, the antipellagra vitamin. The American Medical Association and the American Institute of Nutrition urged the adoption of the new name, niacin, to avoid any suggestion that the B-complex vitamin might be a chemical cousin of nicotine, which it is.

night blindness   The total or partial loss of the ability to see in dim light. In addition to poor vision in dim light, night blindness is also characterized by difficulty of the eyes to adjust to light intensity changes, such as going from a brightly lighted room into one that is relatively dark. The condition is associated with the lack of a visual pigment, *rhodopsin*, in the retinal layer of the eyes. A common cause of the lack of rhodopsin is a deficiency of vitamin A, which is a component of the rhodopsin molecule. Also called *nyctalopia*.

nitrates   Chemicals that are salts formed by the combination of nitric acid with a mineral, such as sodium or potassium. Potassium nitrate is used as an additive in pickling brine and in chopped and cured meats as a color preservative. Sodium nitrate is also used as a color preservative in cured meats, frankfurters, bacon, smoked and spiced ham, and other food products. The nitrates have been a source of controversy because of evidence that they can combine with amines in the digestive tract to form substances called *nitrosamines*, which cause cancer. See *nitrites*.

nitrites   chemicals that are salts produced by the reaction of nitrous acid with a mineral compound, usually one containing potassium or sodium. Both sodium and potassium nitrites are used as color preservatives in processed meats and other food products. In addition to preserving the fresh red color of meats, they help protect foods against the development of bacteria that cause food poisoning, such as botulism. Nitrites can be converted by bacteria to nitrates and nitrates can be converted by plant enzymes to nitrites. Nitrites as well as nitrates can be converted to cancer-causing nitrosamines by combining with amines in foods and other sources in the digestive tract. See *nitrates*.

nitrogen   An inert gas that constitutes about 80 percent of the air in the atmosphere. Nitrogen is also a component of all amino acids, and therefore, of all proteins. The nitrogen content of various plant proteins ranges from about 13 percent in avocados to nearly 20 percent in almonds. In protein metabolism, the nitrogen component is often discarded as it becomes a part of the ammonia-urea step of urine production. Because the nitrogen portion of amino acids cannot be "burned" as body fuel, the caloric value of proteins is about the same as that of sugar, or 4 calories per gram of protein.

nitrogen balance   The relationship between the amount of nitrogen entering the body through food and the amount excreted. A positive nitrogen balance exists when the amount consumed is greater than the amount excreted. A negative nitrogen balance occurs when nitrogen is excreted faster than it is consumed in foods. A negative nitrogen balance can develop if the body is forced to burn amino acids as a source of energy because the diet lacks carbohydrates or fatty acids that can be utilized as fuel. A positive nitrogen balance is normal for individuals who are adding muscle tissue to their body frames, such as growing children or people recovering from illness or injury.

nitrosamines   Chemical compounds formed by the combination of amines and nitrates. They have been found to be a cause of cancer in laboratory animals and are considered a potential source of stomach and other cancers in humans. Nitrosamines have been found in beers and in several brands of Scotch whiskey; they have also been found in air pollution samples. See *nitrates; nitrites*.

nondairy products   Manufactured foods offered as substitutes for milk products for use by people who are allergic to milk components or who wish to avoid milk for religious or other reasons. Nondairy products include coffee whiteners and whipped cream substitutes made from vegetable fats, such as coconut oil. Some nondairy products contain lactose, or milk sugar, and casein, the protein component of milk. Most nondairy products are not true equivalents of milk in terms of nutritional value and critics recommend reading the labels carefully. See *filled milk*.

nonelectrolytes A term sometimes applied to substances in body cells and fluids that do not ionize, or acquire a positive or negative electrical charge. Examples of nonelectrolytes include glucose, proteins, and urea.

nonessential amino acids Amino acids that are not required in proteins consumed because the chemical factories of the human body can manufacture them from other substances in the tissues. One example is alanine, a nonessential amino acid the human body can manufacture from pyruvic acid present in the muscle tissue.

nonnutritive sweeteners Any sugar substitute that does not contribute calories or other nutrients to the food sweetened. Examples of nonnutritive sweeteners include saccharin, cyclamates, and aspartame. Some nonnutritive sweeteners actually contain the same number of calories per measured weight as sugar, 4 calories per gram, but their sweetness is so intense that much smaller amounts are needed and the caloric content is negligible. Aspartame, for example, is 160 times as sweet as sugar, so 1 oz. of aspartame is equivalent to about 11 lb. of sugar.

nonorganic A term sometimes used to identify foods that are not organically grown, in lieu of using a somewhat less meaningful term, like "unnatural food," as distinguished from natural food.

nonprescription drugs See *OTC drugs*.

nonvitamins A term applied to substances that resemble vitamins in their effects on the body, but which have not been proven to be "true" vitamins in the sense that they cannot be manufactured by the body and a deficiency of these substances can lead to specific adverse health effects. Nonvitamins include a variety of substances that may be vitamins for other animals, but not for humans. One example is carnitine, which is required in the diets of certain lower forms of animal life but which occurs naturally in human tissues and is usually not required in human diets. Vitamin C, on the other hand, is required as a true vitamin for humans but it is synthesized by most other animals.

norepinephrine A neurotransmitter substance secreted by the adrenal glands. It is a close chemical relative of epinephrine, but is generally less potent. Epinephrine can be synthesized in the body from norepinephrine; both are manufactured in the body by the metabolism of the amino acid tyrosine.

norleucine A nonessential amino acid that is a component of many proteins and which can also be manufactured as an artificial nutrient. Norleucine occurs naturally in proteins of nerve tissue.

nucleic acid A large, complex, and important substance found in all living cells. Nucleic acids contain phosphoric acid, sugar molecules, and other components that work together to control the general processes of metabolism. They are also involved in many chemical reactions of cell metabolism without becoming a part of the substances that result. Examples of nucleic acids include DNA and RNA.

nutrient Any substance that affects the metabolic processes of the human body. Essential nutrients are substances like amino acids, fatty acids, carbohydrates, minerals, and vitamins that are necessary for normal growth and functioning and the maintenance of life, and which must be supplied by foods because they cannot be manufactured by body tissues. Secondary nutrients are substances that stimulate the "friendly microorganisms" in the body to manufacture other nutrients.

nutrient density See *index of nutritional quality*.

nutrient requirements, adult The recommended dietary allowances, adjusted for age, weight, sex, physical activity, and other individual factors. Although individual requirements may vary from day to day, the RDAs represent an average need with a small amount of reserves for most adults.

nutrient requirements, pregnancy The recommended dietary allowances, adjusted to accommodate an average weight gain of between 20 and 25 lb. over a period of 9 months. Specific dietary factors include a need for foods rich in proteins, vitamins, and minerals, particularly iron and folic acid. During pregnancy, the average mother gains about 6 lb. in increased blood volume and increased size of the uterus and breasts; the fetus, placenta, and amniotic fluid account for about 10 lb. of the weight gain. Part of the remaining weight gain occurs in the form of fat storage about the hips and back.

nutrient supplements A term sometimes applied to the use of vitamin or mineral supplements in food processing, such as the commercial processing of milk where vitamin D is added or the addition of B vitamins during the manufacture of refined flour or rice.

nutrification A term applied to the manufacture of substitute or synthetic foods that are presumed to contain the same nutrients as a real food item. One example could be a meat substitute. If claims are made that the meat substitute contains the same nutrients as real meat, the nutrients must be present and accounted for in proportions equal to or greater than those in the real food.

nutrition The sum total of all the processes involved in eating, assimilating, and utilizing nutrients, including all the mechanisms whereby the body uses food for energy, growth, and maintenance.

nutritional supplements The vitamins and minerals sold in tablet, capsule, or liquid form to supplement the vitamins and minerals in the diet. Nutritional supplements enable persons with special dietary needs to obtain their recommended dietary allowances of vitamins and minerals. Women who are pregnant or who use oral contraceptives often require nutritional supplements, as do vegetarians and others who do not eat meat, eggs, milk, or certain other foods for religious, cultural, or other reasons, or people with food allergies. Others who may require nutritional supplements include cigarette smokers, drinkers of caffeine beverages, and persons subject to psychological stress. See *vitamin supplements; mineral supplements*.

nyctalopia See *night blindness*.

O

obesity An accumulation of fat in the body that is excessive for the person's age, height, sex, and body build. Some doctors consider a person obese if his body weight is 20 percent above the ideal or average for height, body build, and sex. Others consider a 25 percent weight gain as a measure of obesity, pointing out that for a "normal" person up to 25 percent of the body weight is fat. Adding another 25 percent doubles the amount of fat carried on the body frame and justifies identifying the person as obese.

odontoma A medical term for a mouth problem in which a tooth fails to erupt because of a tumor at that point on the gumline.

oleic acid An unsaturated fatty acid found in many plant and animal fats, probably the most widely distributed of all fatty acids. It is the major fatty acid in beef, lamb, pork, poultry, eggs, milk, and butter.

oleoresin An extract of a spice, usually employing alcohol as the solvent, which is later removed by distillation. Oleoresins are used to create a flavor or aroma that is too weak in the natural plant product to be appreciated by a consumer. The oleoresin flavor of a spice may be anywhere from 5 to 20 times as strong as the natural spice flavor.

oral contraceptives A device in the form of a pill containing female sex hormones that controls ovulation in a woman and thereby regulates her menstrual cycle. The contraceptive pill in effect fools the body chemistry into believing an ovum has been released and a pregnancy has been started. This illusion also creates the impression within the body's hormonal system that the next ovum should not be prepared for release. At the end of the normal menstrual cycle, the lining of the uterus is sloughed off as would ordinarily occur. Oral contraceptives can interfere with the absorption of B vitamins, vitamin C, folic acid, and zinc.

organic A term that suggests an organ or organs or organism and which is usually applied when identifying substances that are derived from living organisms. However, it is also used to identify any substance containing carbon or carbon and hydrogen, which are present in most living organisms. See *nonorganic*.

organic gardening Gardening conducted without the use of synthetic chemical fertilizers and pesticides. Manure may be used as a "natural fertilizer, and bugs may be picked by hand from the fruits and vegetables. Although popularized as a method of producing foods free of potentially harmful chemicals for natural or organic food lovers, the method is also used by scientists when attempting to trace the source of cancer-causing substances in agricultural products. Tobacco, for example, may be grown in "virgin" soil without the use of chemical fertilizers or insecticides to determine which chemical, if any, used in commercial tobacco production may be a cause of cancer in cigarette smokers.

organic nutrients A term applied to any essential nutrients obtained from natural food sources, even when extracted from natural foods for use as supplements. The term is also applied to food items grown without the use of chemical fertilizers or pesticides.

orthomolecular therapy An alternative term for megavitamin therapy, particularly when applied to the treatment of mental health disorders associated with vitamin deficiencies. The term was introduced by Dr. Linus Pauling who combined the words *orthodox*, meaning "something that is right and proper," and *molecule*; the combination is intended to identify a practice of getting the proper molecules into the body in the right amounts.

osmosis A force in nature that causes two bodies of fluids containing dissolved substances to flow together so that the concentration of dissolved particles is the same in each body. The process occurs through a membrane that is semipermeable, meaning it appears to be solid but has tiny openings large enough for certain molecules to pass through. The membranes of most tissue cells are semipermeable and osmosis is the process that enables fluids and certain nutrients to pass into and out of the cells.

ossification The formation of bone or the conversion of a substance into bone. Most bones in the body develop by an ossification process in which calcium and other mineral salts are deposited in cartilage structures that are the same general shape as the bones they replace. Even while growing, long bones become longer by the continuous deposit of minerals in the cartilage areas between the shaft and end portions of the bones.

osteomalacia A bone disease that is usually characterized by pain and tenderness and is caused by the failure of new bone to develop normally. It is similar to rickets, which affects the still-growing bones of children, except that osteomalacia occurs in older persons whose bones have already formed. It results from the excretion of bone minerals at a faster rate than they are replaced by the amount of calcium and phosphorus in the diet.

osteoporosis   A bone disease in which there is a loss of minerals from the bones. Like osteomalacia, this disorder is often associated with an inadequate intake of calcium and phosphorus in the diet. However, osteoporosis may also result in part from a lack of physical activity, meaning a disuse of the limbs, and a failure of the body to deposit fresh minerals where it feels they are not needed. The bones eventually become thin and brittle and break easily, sometimes during ordinary activities that put pressure on the weakened bones. The only other symptom may be bone pain.

OTC drugs   A popular name for drugs you can buy at a drugstore or supermarket that do not require a doctor's prescription. The letters stand for *over the counter*. Also called *nonprescription drugs*.

overage   The practice of compensating for the natural loss of potency of a vitamin or other nutrient while it is on a store shelf by adding an extra amount when it is manufactured. Overage is also applied to certain foods that contain vitamins or other essential nutrients.

overdose   A dose of a drug or other substance in excess of what is required for normal function that is likely to cause adverse effects. The difference between a normal dose and an overdose varies with the substance and with the age, size, and general health of the individual.

oxalates   Any of the salts formed by the combination of a mineral with oxalic acid. Oxalates formed in the digestive tract result in binding minerals, such as calcium and magnesium, so they cannot be absorbed through the wall of the small intestine. They may instead be excreted in the urine with the risk of forming kidney stones. About 70 percent of kidney stone cases requiring hospitalization involve oxalic acid salts. See *oxalic acid*.

oxalic acid   An organic acid present in rhubarb, dried apricots, blackberries, blueberries, currants, and certain vegetable greens, such as spinach. Oxalic acid forms a compound, calcium oxalate, with calcium in the digestive tract, causing the calcium to pass through without being absorbed. The amount of calcium lost depends in part on the proportions of calcium and oxalic acid foods in the diet; as more oxalic acid foods are included in meals, the amount of calcium intake must also be increased.

oxidation   A term that literally means the addition of oxygen. In actual chemical processes, the term may also refer to the removal of oxygen—which is transferred to another molecule—or to the removal of hydrogen atoms from a molecule. In food metabolism, oxidation refers to the addition of oxygen to carbon atoms as food molecules are broken down. The process involves the release of energy and the production of carbon dioxide, from the carbon and oxygen reaction, which is released through the lungs when one exhales. Because a nutrient may go through several steps of reactions during metabolism, oxidation and the production of carbon dioxide may occur at each step.

oxygen A colorless, odorless gas that makes up 20 percent of the air we breathe. Oxygen also accounts for 90 percent of the weight of water, which is a combination of oxygen and hydrogen. Oxygen is the most important chemical element in the maintenance of life of most organisms, including humans. A human can live for weeks without food, for days without water, but for only a few minutes without oxygen. Every body cell requires oxygen to continue living and each cell depends on the flow of oxygen in the bloodstream; when blood flow is interrupted by a blocked artery or a ruptured blood vessel, it is the loss of oxygen that accounts for the symptoms of heart attack or stroke or similar effects. Most of the chemical reactions of metabolism involve the use of oxygen. When a carbohydrate is metabolized, for example, about 1 qt. of oxygen is required to burn each gram of carbohydrate; since the air is only 20 percent oxygen, one has to inhale 5 qt. of air for each gram of carbohydrate metabolized. To release the energy in 1 oz. of fat, a person has to inhale about 300 qt. of air. See *infarction; ischemia; oxidation; oxygen debt*.

oxygen debt A term that refers to the "borrowing" of oxygen from body stores, mainly in the muscle tissues, during vigorous exercise. When the physical exertion has ended, and often before, the individual spends several minutes huffing and puffing to repay the oxygen debt. The oxygen acquired during the period of heavy breathing is actually needed for the oxidation of lactic acid, which is a by-product of the burning of glucose during muscle contractions. Because glucose is burned faster than lactic acid can be oxidized during vigorous exercise, the lactic acid accumulates until the body can play "oxygen catch-up." Also called *second wind*.

oxystearin A modified fatty acid that occurs as a tan, waxy substance in animal fats. It is used as a crystallization inhibitor in vegetable oils, preventing a cloudy appearance in the oils at low temperatures. Oxystearin is also used as a defoaming agent in yeast and sugar beet processing and as a coating for pills.

oxytetracycline An antibiotic used as an additive in poultry processing. Oxytetracycline may be added to the feed of turkeys and chickens to stimulate growth. Their carcasses are later dipped in oxytetracycline to retard the development of a rancid flavor.

ozone A molecule of oxygen that contains three oxygen atoms instead of the usual two. It may appear as a bluish gas or liquid which has antiseptic and disinfectant powers. However, it is also irritating and toxic to the human respiratory system. Ozone occurs in areas of air pollution and is responsible for the smell in the air from an electrical discharge, such as a lightning strike. Ozone is used commercially as a water purifier and bleaching agent.

P

PABA See *para-aminobenzoic acid*.

pagophagia A medical term for ice-eating. People who crave ice usually suffer from iron-deficiency anemia and many give up ice-eating when provided with iron supplements. It is not unusual for a pagophagia patient to consume several trays of ice cubes in a day. See *pica*.

pangamic acid A substance promoted as vitamin B-15 and reportedly composed of sodium gluconate, glycine, and other substances. The U.S. Food and Drug Administration has challenged the claims of the manufacturer that the substance is a vitamin or has any therapeutic value. Pangamic acid, it has been claimed, provides relief from arthritis, nerve pain, asthma, and skin disorders.

pantothenic acid A vitamin that is a part of the vitamin B-complex. It occurs in all living tissues of plants and animals, playing a role in the metabolism of fats and carbohydrates. It also serves as a growth substance for certain organisms, such as yeast.

The name of the vitamin is derived from the Greek word *pantos*, meaning "all" or "everywhere," because pantothenic acid is so widely distributed in nature that a deficiency is unusual. However, through experiments with animals and human volunteers, it has been found that a diet from which pantothenic acid has been excluded results in depressed metabolism of fats and carbohydrates. Chickens and rats deprived of pantothenic acid develop a skin disease that is cured when the vitamin is restored to their diets. Humans fed meals lacking pantothenic acid reported feelings of nausea, abdominal distress, muscle cramps, fatigue, headaches, insomnia, feelings of numbness and tingling in the hands and feet, loss of coordination, and personality changes. Again, the complaints disappeared when pantothenic acid was restored to their experimental diets. One surprising result of feeding pantothenic-acid–deficient diets to monkeys, dogs, and other animals was premature graying of the hair.

The vitamin is available in most foods, although some items, such as liver, eggs, yeast, wheat germ, peas, and peanuts, are better than others. Except for broccoli and sweet potatoes, most fruits and vegetable sources contain small amounts of pantothenic acid. It is also easily available in vitamin supplements. Nutrition experts have found that prolonged cooking or heating of foods can destroy pantothenic acid, which is also an integral part of the coenzyme A needed to synthesize certain adrenal hormones.

para-aminobenzoic acid A substance that is a component of folic acid. It is sometimes included in lists of vitamins, although its status is controversial and para-aminobenzoic acid itself is not considered an essential element in the human diet. It is used in medications to treat rickettsial diseases and in preparations used on the skin to prevent sunburn. Abbreviated *PABA*.

parathormone A hormone of the parathyroid, a gland next to the thyroid. It regulates the amount of calcium moving into and out of bones. Vitamin D is important in this activity.

parathyroid hormone A hormone secreted by the parathyroid glands, which are located in pairs beside the thyroid glands. It regulates the metabolism of calcium and phosphorus in the body. Calcium levels are controlled directly by monitoring the level of calcium ions in the blood; when the calcium ion level drops below a minimum, the parathyroid hormone signals the removal of calcium from the bones. Levels of phosphorus are regulated indirectly through the calcium-phosphorus balance system of the body. The function of the parathyroid glands has been known only since 1900. Prior to that, these glands were often removed during thyroid surgery and the patient subsequently died from parathyroid hormone deficiency symptoms.

partially incomplete protein A classification of a protein that can sustain life, but does not support growth because of a missing essential amino acid. Gliadin, a wheat protein lacking in lysine, is one example. See *incomplete protein*.

pasteurization The process of heating milk or other fluids to kill certain disease-causing bacteria and retard the development of others. The fluid is usually heated to a temperature of 140°F (60°C) for a period of 30 min. The process is named for Louis Pasteur, a nineteenth-century French doctor, who was a pioneer in the study of methods of preventing bacteria-spoiled food.

patch test A technique for testing the reaction of a person to a possible allergen by placing a sample of the substance on the inner surface of an adhesive bandage and fastening the bandage to the patient's skin. After 24 to 48 hr., a skin reaction reaction under the bandage will indicate whether the person is allergic to the substance.

pectin   A carbohydrate molecule found in the cell walls and other structural components of plants. The pectin used in jellies and jams is obtained from citrus peel and apple peel and cores that have been dried, then boiled in water for about 40 min. The heat and acids in the fruit material result in a substance that will help form a gel in the presence of a strong sugar concentration. The gel provides the semisolid material of jellies and jams.

pellagra   A vitamin-deficiency disease with signs and symptoms that involve the skin, mind, and digestive tract. The cause may be a lack of niacin in the diet or the inability to convert the amino acid tryptophan into niacin. In pellagra, the skin becomes thick and red, especially on the hands and arms. Untreated, the skin becomes cracked and a source of infection. Mental symptoms vary from insomnia and depression to violent, irrational behavior. Vomiting, diarrhea, and loss of appetite are among the digestive disorders. Symptoms diminish when niacin or foods rich in this B vitamin are administered to a pellagra patient.

pepsin   An enzyme that is the chief digestive component of the stomach's gastric juice. Pepsin acts on certain proteins in foods, particularly those in which tyrosine or phenylalanine are components of the protein molecule. Pepsin also has some milk-clotting action similar to that of rennin.

peptic ulcers   An ulceration of the digestive tract caused by the erosion of the mucous membrane lining anywhere from the lower esophagus to the duodenum due to the action of the highly acid gastric juice of the stomach. Peptic ulcers are usually identified according to their location, such as gastric ulcers (in the stomach) or duodenal ulcers (in the duodenum). Peptic ulcers can affect men and women of all ages, races, and occupations, although men who are subject to stress are the usual candidates. Treatment includes medication, diet, and surgery.

pesticide residues in food   The poisonous substances that accumulate in the food chain from many decades of spraying agricultural and residential areas with insect killers and applying other poisons in food storage areas to kill rodents and other vermin. A federal law passed in 1954 established a zero tolerance level, meaning no traces of pesticides would be permitted on foods sold. However, it is virtually impossible to produce foods that have not been exposed to at least one of the pesticides that has entered the soil, water, or air since the end of World War II. Pesticides tend to accumulate in greater concentrations in meats, particularly fatty meats, because pesticides like DDT tend to be absorbed by fats.

pH A bit of chemical shorthand that stands for the hydrogen ion concentration of a substance and indicates its degree of acidity or alkalinity. A pH of 7 is regarded as neutral. Numbers that are lower than 7 are considered acid and those higher than 7 are alkaline, or base, on the pH scale. The lower the pH number, the greater the degree of acidity. The pH numbers run from 0 to 14, with 14 the rating of the most alkaline substance possible.

phenylalanine An essential amino acid required for normal growth in infants and nitrogen equilibrium in adults. Phenylalanine can be converted by the body's chemistry into a second amino acid, tyrosine; the two are often considered together because one is the precursor of the other. Phenylalanine is involved in the production of melanin, the pigment responsible for skin color, and is glucogenic, meaning it can be a source of glucose via metabolic breakdown processes. In addition, phenylalanine is concerned with the formation of hormones, such as thyroxine, and neurotransmitters like epinephrine and dopamine.

phenylketonuria An inherited disorder that is an inborn error of metabolism caused by the lack of the enzyme necessary to convert the essential amino acid phenylalanine into a second amino acid, tyrosine. As a result, phenylalanine accumulates in the blood. A number of problems, including mental retardation, tremors, poor muscular coordination, and excessive sweating can follow if the disorder is not corrected in early infancy. It can be detected in the first few days of life through a test of the baby's urine, called the *diaper test*. Because tyrosine is involved in the formation of skin pigmentation, a phenylketonuria patient usually has defective skin pigmentation. Abbreviated *PKU*. See *phenylalanine*.

phospholipid A lipid or fatty substance that contains phosphorus. In addition to phosphorus, a phospholipid usually contains two fatty acids, glycerin, and a nitrogen compound. Phospholipids are important because they are involved in the production of hormones and in vital metabolic processes, such as energy release. Lecithin is an example of a phospholipid. Other phospholipids vary according to the kinds of fatty acids they contain.

phosphorus A mineral essential for normal human health that is utilized in a variety of phosphate compounds rather than as a pure element. About 1 percent of human body weight is phosphorus, most of it combined with calcium in the structure of bones and teeth. The remainder is involved in the metabolic activities of proteins, fats, and carbohydrates, in particular as part of an energy-rich molecule, adenosine triphosphate (ATP), that plays a significant role in providing power for muscle contractions.

It is believed that at least a few molecules of phosphates can be found in every one of the body's trillions of tissue cells. Phosphorus is closely associated with calcium in body functions and the body normally maintains a ratio between the two minerals. Both are absorbed from the intestine in an acid medium with the help of vitamin D; an abnormal balance of calcium:phosphorus interferes with the absorption of both minerals. Factors that impair phosphorus absorption include the use of antacid medications and high dietary levels of other minerals, such as iron, that combine with phosphorus to form insoluble phosphate compounds.

Food sources that have high protein levels are good sources of phosphorus, whose distribution in nature seems to follow proteins. Meat, fish, poultry, eggs, milk, cheese, nuts, and legumes are among the best food sources. Cereal grains contain phosphorus, but it is usually bound in phytic acid and cannot be absorbed by the body. A deficiency of phosphorus is rare, but it can result from abuse of antacid medications and is characterized by loss of minerals and softening of the bones.

phylloquinone   An alternate term for *vitamin K*. See this entry.

physical stress   The change that may come in the physiological demand for calories and nutrients in an individual during heavy labor, physical exertion, strenuous athletics, or because of environmental conditions.

physiological stress   Any additional metabolic demands placed on the body, such as occur in fever, illness, surgery, or infection. Pregnancy and lactation, although normal processes for females, are considered to place a physiological stress on the individual.

phytic acid   An organic acid found in the bran portion of cereals. Phytic acid tends to bind with calcium in the intestine to form insoluble salts, thereby making the calcium unavailable for absorption from the digestive tract. Meals that contain large amounts of bran or whole cereals can adversely affect the ability of the body to absorb calcium, unless large amounts of calcium-rich foods are eaten to compensate for the proportion lost by acid binding.

pica   A craving for abnormal foods or food substitutes. The individual usually eats only one kind of unnatural food, which may be laundry starch, paint, clay, or dirt. Pica is believed to be caused by a nutritional deficiency, such as iron-deficiency anemia. Ice-eating, called *pagophagia*, is a form of pica that usually can be treated by giving the person iron supplements. The term may also be applied to cases of pregnant women who develop cravings for strange foods.

piles   See *hemorrhoids*.

peptide   Any substance composed of two or more amino acids. A peptide is often identified by the number of amino acids it contains, such as *dipeptide* for two amino acids, *tripeptide* for three amino acids, and so on.

pernicious anemia A form of anemia in which the digestive tract is unable to absorb vitamin B-12 from the small intestine because of the absence of a substance, the *intrinsic factor*, normally produced by cells lining the stomach. The B-12 vitamin is required for the production of red blood cells. It is also necessary for a healthy nervous system, so pernicious anemia is often associated with neurological disorders. The condition usually develops around middle age in people whose ancestry is of northwestern Europe. However, there is a lack of evidence that the disorder is hereditary.

placebo Any medication given to relieve symptoms, even though it does not contain any active drugs and depends solely on psychological effects for its function. A placebo may be administered by a doctor who can find no organic cause for the complaints of a patient. Placebo substances may also be used in human experiments in which one-half the subjects of a test are given a real drug and the other half a pill or capsule that looks like the drug, but contains only starch or sugar or some other harmless substance. Only the person conducting the experiment would know which pills were placebos and which were real drugs. Also called *dummy*.

placenta An organ that develops during pregnancy as a link between the lining of the mother's uterus and the developing offspring. The placenta is actually composed of two parts, a uterine part for the mother and a fetal part for the offspring. The placenta allows nutrients from the mother's blood to diffuse into the blood of the fetus and the waste products from the fetus to diffuse back into the mother's blood to be excreted. A semipermeable membrane separates the two parts of the placenta and serves as a filter that allows some materials to pass through while others are screened out. Also called *afterbirth*.

plaque A deposit of foreign material on the surface of a body tissue. Examples include the plaques of fatty material that accumulate on the lining of arteries in atheroslcerosis and accumulation of foreign material on the surface of a tooth, which is called *dental plaque*, or *bacterial plaque* because it harbors the bacteria that cause tooth decay. The accumulation of plaque on artery walls contributes to coronary heart disease when it becomes so thick that it narrows the opening through which blood can flow.

polymer A chemical compound formed by the union of several or more smaller chemical compounds, which may be called *monomers*. The monomers may or may not be different. Examples of polymers include starches and celluloses, which are large molecules composed of a number of simple sugar molecules.

polyunsaturated fats and oils Food fats that contain polyunsaturated fatty acids, such as linoleic acid, and which tend to become rancid in the presence of oxygen. Cottonseed, corn, and soybean oils contain polyunsaturated fatty acids. Polyunsaturated fats that break down in reactions with oxygen molecules in the air account for much of the rancid flavor of peanuts, potato chips, and other products that become stale quickly when exposed to the air. See *polyunsaturated fatty acids*.

polyunsaturated fatty acids Fatty acids that consist of chains of carbon atoms with two or more points in the chain where hydrogen atoms can be added. The terms *saturated* and *unsaturated* refer to the degree of saturation of the molecule with hydrogen atoms. A saturated fatty acid cannot hold any additional hydrogen atoms but an unsaturated fatty acid can accommodate one more, whereas a polyunsaturated acid can hold several more. Examples of polyunsaturated fatty acids include linoleic, linolenic, and arachidonic acids. A fatty acid generally becomes more solid and less fluid as it becomes saturated. Thus, liquid vegetable oils are usually rich in polyunsaturated fatty acids. Abbreviated *PUFA*.

porphyrins A group of related substances derived from the amino acid glycine and involved in the respiration of plant and animal tissues. Of particular importance to human respiration is a porphyrin that contains the mineral iron. It is known as *heme*, and when combined with a certain protein it becomes hemoglobin, the red oxygen-carrying pigment of the red blood cells.

postlateral sclerosis The name of a disease caused by a nutritional deficiency that results in degeneration of the spinal cord. This deficiency disease is caused by a lack of the *intrinsic factor*, which combines with the *extrinsic factor* to form vitamin B-12. It is marked by a loss of myelin in certain nerves of the spinal cord, resulting in a loss of feeling in the arms and legs, confusion and mental changes, and muscle wasting. Untreated, the disease is often fatal within 2 years, but with vitamin B-12 treatment good health can be maintained indefinitely.

potassium A chemical element and essential mineral in human nutrition. All body cells, but particularly the muscle cells, require high levels of potassium. It is very important for normal heart function, in maintaining an acid-base balance, and in helping to regulate the body's water balance.

Although sodium is the dominant mineral in extracellular fluids, potassium is the important mineral within the cell walls. And where sodium is concentrated in the plasma of the blood, potassium is concentrated in the red blood cells. Potassium occurs in many types of food and deficiencies of potassium are rare, except as a result of diarrhea, prolonged intravenous feeding, or the use of drugs, such as diuretics, that tend to deplete the body's potassium reserves.

The average North American diet provides about 1 g. of potassium for each 1,000 calories of food intake, which is close to the body's daily needs. Symptoms of a potassium deficiency include muscular weakness, mental disorientation, increased nervous irritability, and heart, digestive, and breathing problems. Good food sources of potassium include cocoa and instant coffee, whole-grain cereal products, milk, most meats and fish, legumes, nuts, sorghum molasses, and most vegetables. Eggs, cheese, fruits, and fats are among the poor sources of potassium.

potassium chloride   A chemical compound of potassium and chlorine used as a table salt substitute for persons on low sodium diets. Potassium chloride is also used as an electrolyte source that can be administered orally or intravenously for patients suffering electrolyte loss due to illness or injury. See *salt substitutes*.

preservative   Any chemical or process designed to increase the safety of a food product by protecting it and the consumer from the hazards of spoilage and food poisoning while extending the life of the taste, aroma, and other freshness qualities of the food. Chemical preservatives include those that kill or retard the growth of microorganisms or that prevent enzyme or oxidation effects which may result in rancidity or other adverse changes in edibility. Preservative processes include freezing and the use of heat, as in *pasteurization*. See this entry.

proband   A person who is the basis for a study of a possible genetic or family disorder. For example, if a person shows signs of an inborn error of metabolism, he becomes the proband of a study to determine whether any blood relatives show the same signs or symptoms.

processed foods   Foods that have been dried, canned, frozen, treated with additives or preservatives, irradiated, or otherwise altered from their original qualities of freshness. Food processing is generally necessary to ensure a year-round supply of fruits, vegetables, and other food products that would otherwise be available in quantity only during a brief period of the year. However, any processing method reduces the nutritional value of most foods. Frozen fruits and vegetables retain less than 85 percent of the nutritional quality they had when fresh, whereas canned fruits and vegetables may retain only about 60 percent of their original nutritional value.

proline   A nonessential amino acid found in the protein molecules of collagen, a structural tissue of skin, tendons, and bone. The conversion of the amino acid into the form used by the body in producing collagen requires the presence of vitamin C, or ascorbic acid. In a case of scurvy, or vitamin C deficiency, proline is not incorporated into collagen and the connective tissue produced by the body is defective. The slow healing of wound and burn injuries in scurvy victims results from the faulty proline conversion process, which also accounts for other symptoms of *scurvy*. See this entry.

prostaglandins A group of hormone-like substances produced naturally from fatty acids and capable of causing effects on the metabolic, circulatory, nervous, and female reproductive systems. Prostaglandins were first found in human semen and given a name suggesting that the prostate gland was the source. Later research showed prostaglandins are produced by many tissues of numerous kinds of organisms. There are four basic kinds of prostaglandins, each with several variations. The prostaglandin source in most cases is arachidonic fatty acid, which in turn is derived from linoleic acid in the diet.

protein efficiency ratio A measure of protein quality established by the U.S. Food and Drug Administration. The efficiency ratio of a protein is determined in laboratory tests in which rats are fed a protein food for 28 days and their weight gain is compared to a similar group of rats fed casein, or milk protein. The ratio is then calculated according to a mathematical formula. If the protein tested has a value less than 20 percent that of casein (a ratio of 2.5 according to the formula), it must be identified on a label as "not a significant source of protein." Abbreviated *PER*.

protein hydrolysate A medical formulation of essential and nonessential amino acids and minerals prescribed for patients who require a special build-up of body tissues as a result of a serious illness or as part of preoperative or postoperative therapy. The nutrients, which can be administered by injection or in tablet form, provide source material for the body's own tissue-building mechanisms. Amino acid-mineral complexes are also administered by intravenous injection for patients whose digestive tracts cannot handle protein foods in the normal manner.

protein isolates Highly purified proteins isolated from oil-free, food-protein concentrates, such as soybean, cottonseed, and sesame.

protein-rich mixtures Mixtures high in protein from sources like peanuts, skim milk, soya, corn, wheat, and legumes, with added minerals and vitamins. One example is corn-soy-milk.

proteins Any of a large group of organic compounds containing carbon, hydrogen, nitrogen, and oxygen and generally composed of long chains of amino acids including those elements. They are essential components of nuclei and protoplasm as well as most extracellular fluids of animals. Proteins often occur as very large and complex molecules built from thousands of amino acid units. But, regardless of size and structure, all proteins have in common an amino group, consisting of a nitrogen atom attached to two hydrogen atoms, and a carboxyl group, which contains a carbon and hydrogen atom separated by two oxygen atoms.

   The properties of the various proteins are determined by the quantity and quality of the amino acids and the manner in which they are arranged in the protein molecule. A linkage of two amino acids is called a *dipeptide*, a peptide being a constituent part of a protein; a linkage of many amino acids is a *polypeptide*. Because the chain of amino acids in a protein, or polypeptide, can have almost any number of side chains, various proteins can exist in the shape of long chains, spirals, baskets, or hollow spheres. Also, since the constituent amino acids can be acidic or alkaline, so can the protein.

A protein can form a chemical bond with a fat to become a *lipoprotein*, with a carbohydrate to become a *glucoprotein*, or with a mineral, such as iron. In fact, the red coloring matter of blood, hemoglobin, is a complex molecule uniting a protein with iron. Proteins containing sulfur or phosphorus are quite common in body tissues.

Proteins are usually associated with muscle tissue, probably because of the dependence of most North Americans on meat as a source of proteins. However, proteins are also found in blood cells, as noted previously, and also in enzymes, hormones, connective tissue, membranes, antibodies, blood-clotting components, and albumin. In the absence of carbohydrates and fats, protein can be converted by the body's chemical factories to glucose molecules. During a period of starvation, or even during a crash diet, the body muscles may be stripped of the amino acid alanine, which is easily converted to glucose to stoke the body's furnaces. The average human body can lose protein at a rate of about 2 oz. per day for a short period of time before irreversible damage and possible death occur. The average adult body contains between 17 and 26 lb. of protein, which represents as much as 48,000 calories of potential fuel at 4 calories per gram of protein. But only a fraction of the body's protein could be self-digested during a period of starvation before the body systems would be rendered useless by the very process of trying to remain alive by burning protein molecules.

The average North American diet provides about 400 calories, or 100 g., per day in protein. The amount actually ranges between about 70 and 125 g. for most normal adults. People with certain disease conditions, particularly kidney diseases, may have much lower protein intakes because the nitrogen excreted during protein metabolism can be an added burden to diseased kidneys. For most individuals, protein quality is more important than protein quantity because at least 13 g. of protein consumed each day should consist of the essential amino acids. As described elsewhere, essential amino acids are required by the body in the foods eaten because the body cannot manufacture its own. Essential amino acids are available in a variety of foods, but certain proteins called *complete proteins* are better sources than others. The reason they are called complete proteins is that they contain all the essential amino acids. The list is fairly short and consists primarily of eggs and milk. Because eggs and milk represent nature's way of starting and sustaining animal life, it seems reasonable that nature would ensure that the egg and infant nourishment should be as nearly a complete nutritional package as possible. However, many adults cannot live on milk and eggs alone, and other combinations of essential amino acids must be found.

Other foods that contain the essential amino acids, though in smaller amounts than eggs and milk, include wheat germ, corn germ, meat, fish, soybeans, whole rice, casein, whole wheat, potatoes, wheat gluten, whole oats, barley, brewer's yeast, whole corn, whole rye, buckwheat, peanuts, and dried beans and peas. Other vegetable products contain some but not all of the essential amino acids, but by combining them properly it is possible to create a meal that is entirely vegetarian and supplies all of the amino acids. The catch is making a combination of grains, legumes, or other vegetables that contain all the essential amino acids without also adding excessive calories or an imbalance of other nutrients at the same time.

It has been demonstrated by nutrition experts that it is possible to prepare a diet that contains all the essential amino acids from fruits and vegetables, but divided into three meals per day the vegetarian must eat over 3 lb. of food and consume 2,000 calories at each meal. To get the same amount of protein contained in a 3-oz. serving of meat, one would have to eat 1 cup of cooked soybeans or 1½ cups of cooked peas. Similarly, to get the same amount of protein as one egg, one would have to eat ½ cup of lima beans or ¾ cup of green peas. Vegetables are a good source of vitamins and minerals and, as noted before, they can be a source of protein. However, it is often easier to get one's daily protein requirements from meat, eggs, and milk—which may be the reason that animal foods are more likely to appear on the tables of more affluent families, sometimes at the expense of a bulk-deficient diet.

In measuring one's daily protein intake in terms of meat, milk, or other sources, it should be remembered that most natural foods, like the human body itself, are mainly water. Muscle meats may be 75 to 80 percent water. As a result, a serving of meat that weighs 100 g., or a little more than 3 oz., may provide no more than 25 g. of protein, and much less if the meat also contains fat. An 8-oz. glass of milk contains slightly more than 1 g. of protein per ounce of fluid. A slice of bread, a medium-size potato, or a 6-oz. cup of oatmeal are worth about 2 g. of protein each, whereas 1 oz. of cheddar cheese or an average egg will provide about 7 g. of protein apiece.

Protein deficiency is one of the most common forms of malnutrition throughout the world. A deficiency of protein, or of one or more of the essential amino acids, may manifest itself in the form of tissue wasting, diarrhea, and fluid accumulation in the abdomen. In Third World countries with protein-deficient diets a disease called *kwashiorkor* often occurs, marked by a skin rash, weakness, anemia, nervous irritability, fatty infiltration of the liver, a loss of ability to digest food normally, and a change in hair color to a reddish-orange shade. Because protein foods are a prime source of B vitamins, a deficiency of the vitamins also results.

protein-sparing action   The process by which fats and carbohydrates, if supplied in the diet in sufficient amounts to meet caloric needs, will spare protein so that it can be used for protein metabolism. When caloric intake is inadequate, protein is used as a source of calories.

prothrombin A substance formed from carbohydrate and protein molecules with the help of vitamin K; it is a necessary component of the normal blood-clotting process. Prothrombin is converted into thrombin in the second stage of blood clotting, after blood platelets have released substances that begin fibrin formation. A deficiency of vitamin K can interfere with this phase of blood clotting. Prothrombin efficiency is tested with blood samples taken from a patient to determine whether the conversion from prothrombin to thrombin is complete and how long the process takes. Also called *clotting factor II*. See *vitamin K; blood clotting*.

provitamin A substance that can be converted into a vitamin by the metabolic mechanisms of the body. One example is beta-carotene, one of the natural pigments found in fruits and vegetables, which is converted in the human intestine into vitamin A. See *carotenes; vitamin A*.

psoriasis A chronic, recurrent skin disease characterized by the appearance of bright red papules and plaques covered with silvery scales. The condition, which is believed to be hereditary, may be complicated by rheumatoid arthritis. Symptoms begin between ages 10 and 40 in most cases and, with the exception of disabling arthritis in some patients, does not affect the general health, although the patient may experience psychological problems because of the appearance of the skin. Some studies have indicated that symptoms of psoriasis may be relieved with vitamin A treatments in addition to other types of therapy, including coal tar and ultraviolet light exposure.

psychological stress Emotional factors that affect appetite, digestion, and utilization of nutrients.

ptomaine poisoning A rare type of food poisoning caused by the products of decomposition of proteins. Although many people identify any food poisoning as ptomaine poisoning, a true case of ptomaine poisoning is unlikely. Ptomaines are potentially poisonous substances produced by bacteria that render proteins putrid, and most people would not eat decomposed meat. Also, most ptomaines, even if they could be eaten, would be converted to relatively harmless substances by the digestive juices of the stomach and intestine. See *food poisoning*.

pull date The date, usually stamped on a food product, that is the last day the food should be offered for sale. Many dairy and meat products carry pull dates. The pull date is based on an estimate of the shelf life of the food when refrigerated in a certain type of package. However, if the product is not kept refrigerated all the time, the pull date can be misleading to the consumer.

Pure Food and Drug Act A law passed by the U.S. Congress in 1938 and modified many times since then that gives the U.S. Food and Drug Administration authority to fine and imprison companies and their personnel for the adulteration and misbranding of food products. Because cosmetics are under the jurisdiction of the FDA, the law also applies to manufacturers and sellers of cosmetics, which often use the same additives as foods and drugs.

purine-free diet A diet designed mainly for gout patients who suffer from a build-up of uric acid and its salts that accumulate in bone joints and cause severe pain. Purine-rich foods are primary sources of uric acid in the blood. They include meat, poultry, and fish, but particularly organ meats, such as liver, kidney, and sweetbreads. They are replaced in the diet by milk, eggs, cheese, and vegetable sources of proteins.

purines A class of organic chemical compounds composed of carbon, hydrogen, and nitrogen that are converted into uric acid when metabolized by the body's chemistry. Two purines, adenine and guanine, are present in nucleic acid molecules, such as DNA. Certain foods are particularly rich in purines and are omitted in purine-free diets. They include anchovies, kidney, liver, meat extracts, sardines, and sweetbreads. Purine-free diets are used by people afflicted with gout who must reduce the sources of uric acid. See *gout*.

purpura A disease marked by bleeding under the skin and through the mucous membranes. Symptoms include the easy development of bruises and small red patches in the skin. There are two types of purpura, *idiopathic* or *primary*, for which the cause is unknown, and *secondary*, which means it is associated with some other disorder, such as anemia, leukemia, rubella, or reactions to drugs or other chemicals. Because purpura is associated with collagen and coagulation disorders, vitamins C and K have been suggested as substances that can relieve symptoms. Malabsorption syndromes that interfere with vitamin uptake may also be linked to symptoms of purpura.

pyridoxal One of three forms of vitamin B-6, the others being pyridoxine and pyridoxamine. Like pyridoxamine, pyridoxal is found in animal food sources and is not as resistant to heat and light as the vegetable form of the vitamin, *pyridoxine*. See this entry.

pyridoxamine The name of one of the three active forms of vitamin B-6. Pyridoxamine is obtained from animal food sources and it is less stable than pyridoxine, a form of the vitamin found in plant food sources. Pyridoxamine is sensitive to light and heat, and cooked meats usually have lost 50 percent of the vitamin. See *pyridoxine; pyridoxal*.

pyridoxine The chemical name of one of the forms of vitamin B-6, a member of the B-complex of water-soluble vitamins. Pyridoxine is the most stable of the different forms of vitamin B-6 and is found mainly in plant food sources; the other forms, pyridoxal and pyridoxamine, occur mainly in animal tissues. However, one form may be converted into another form during metabolic processes.

Pyridoxine was discovered in the 1930s by scientists seeking the cause and cure of a skin disorder. A deficiency of vitamin B-6 causes, among other symptoms, a type of skin disease marked by oily lesions that appear around the mouth and eyes. Other symptoms include nausea, vomiting, dizziness, weight loss, kidney stones, irritability, confusion, and convulsions, most of which respond rapidly to treatment with vitamin B-6.

One of the functions of pyridoxine is the conversion of the amino acid tryptophan into niacin, so that a deficiency of pyridoxine results in the excretion of abnormal breakdown products of tryptophan metabolism. By analyzing the chemicals in a urine sample, medical laboratory technicians can tell whether a person has a pyridoxine deficiency. About 20 different steps in amino acid metabolism require pyridoxine, or the related forms of B-6. Most of the steps involve shifting amino acid groups to form new amino acid molecules and the removal of carbon dioxide from the remaining portions of amino acids. It is also involved in the metabolism of polyunsaturated fatty acids.

The major sources of pyridoxine are muscle and organ meats and whole-grain cereals. Processed foods are generally poor sources. The milling of white flour, for example, removes about three-fourths of its vitamin B-6 content. See *pyridoxal; pyridoxamine.*

pyrosis See *heartburn.*

q

quack A term applied to a person who misrepresents his qualifications and that of his product or services, as in the example of an individual who promotes the use of certain foods or nutrients as cures for various diseases or ailments when there is no scientific evidence to support those claims.

quadriceps The name of a group of four muscles that work together to extend the leg. The muscles extend from the thigh to the lower leg. The name is derived from two Latin words: *quad*, meaning "four," and *a caput*, meaning "head," or, quite literally, "a muscle with four heads."

quality grading A method of sorting agricultural products so that items of a desired maturity are automatically separated from others. A number of products, from peas to coffee beans, are separated by floating them in a water trough, which in some cases may contain salt water to produce a certain density of water and therefore floatability of the item. In quality grading of lima beans, the water density is adjusted so that older beans sink to the bottom while the younger beans of better quality float on top.

quick-energy foods A name given to foods that are claimed to provide energy within a few minutes after being ingested. These claims are controversial—some nutrition experts contend that although the blood sugar level may rise within 30 min after a meal, even candy and cookies require several hours to complete the trip from the mouth to the bloodstream. Certain liquid products that contain mainly glucose and mineral salts similar to those found in body fluids may give added energy in 30 to 60 min; however, much of the quick-energy lift reported by quick-energy food users is believed to be a psychological effect.

quick freezing A method of preserving foods by freezing that was introduced in North America in the 1920s. The difference between quick freezing and ordinary freezing of food is that quick freezing requires that the temperature of the food fall from 32 to 25°F (or −4°C) within 30 min. Because most foods, including meats, contain water with dissolved substances, the actual freezing point of food is several degrees below that of ordinary ice at 32°F (or 0°C).

quinic acid A type of fruit acid found mainly in young peaches, pears, and apples. In mature apples, quinic acid is generally replaced by malic acid. Plums, prunes, and cranberries contain large amounts of quinic acid, which increases the acidity of the urine after it has been converted to benzoic and hippuric acids through metabolism.

quinine A substance obtained from the cinchona tree and used primarily as a medication in the treatment of malaria and muscle cramps. Quinine is also used in beverage formulations for its bitter flavor, particularly in alcoholic beverages like rum and vermouth. It is also a common constituent of bitters. Quinine extract, also known as *cinchona extract*, may be used with certain citrus and other fruit flavors in ice creams and candies.

quinones The name of a group of substances that are the cause of the brown color that appears on certain fruits and vegetables after they have been cut open. Although quinones have no distinctive color of their own, they react readily with other substances in plant foods and with oxygen in the air. The quinone effect not only results in an off-color but leads to the development of off-flavors in foods.

r

rancidity The change in odor and flavor of a fatty substance caused by oxidation processes. A rancid effect may occur in certain vegetables, such as carrots, and the pepper spices, such as paprika, which contain small amounts of fatty acids. The odors of rancid fats are somewhat distinctive. The solid fats of beef and mutton develop the aroma of tallow when rancid, and pork, fish, and some vegetable oils acquire a smell resembling linseed oil. Other vegetable oils and fats from some seafood have a perfume-like odor when rancid. Color changes may also accompany rancidity, usually as a shift to a lighter or bleached shade of the color of the food.

RDA See *recommended dietary allowances*; see also *U.S. RDA* (United States Recommended Daily Allowances).

recall A procedure established by the U.S. Food and Drug Aministration to help retrieve food items from wholesale and retail distribution centers when it has been found that a food product may be hazardous to the health of the consumer. For example, the health hazard might be the presence of botulism in a canned fish product. Recall procedures are rated as Class I, Class II, and Class III, depending on the urgency of the problem. A Class I priority is assigned a product that presents a serious and immediate health threat. Other classes of recall are for less serious health threats. Class III recalls may cover mislabeled foods.

recommended dietary allowances A set of guidelines established by the Food and Nutrition Board of the National Research Council to assist consumers in planning an intake of nutrients that should help a person in good health maintain an adequate state of nutrition. The point about "good health" is important because the recommended dietary allowances may be inadequate for an individual who is afflicted with a debilitating illness or one who is recovering from a serious disease or injury. Also, it should be noted that the recommended dietary allowances do not provide for nutrients lost in the processing of foods or the preparation of foods after they are purchased at the store. Studies show that fruits and vegetables lose between 15 and nearly 40 percent of the nutrients they possessed when fresh by the processes of canning, freezing, and drying. After they are brought home, foods often lose additional nutritional value in cooking, particularly when they are fried. Vitamins like pyridoxamine lose as much as 50 percent of their potency when exposed to the heat of cooking temperatures. Abbreviated *RDA*.

red tongue See *glossitis*.

reducing diet Any diet designed to result in a loss of body weight. Most reducing diets simply curtail the number of calories consumed per day so that for each 3,500 calories of food eliminated from meals 1 lb. of body fat is lost. Reducing diets must be planned carefully so that weight loss is gradual and essential nutrients are not eliminated from meals that have been planned to contain fewer calories.

refined cereal A form of cereal grain that consists primarily of the starchy portion after the outer layers containing the vitamins and minerals have been removed.

refined sugar The term usually applied to ordinary table sugar, which consists of sucrose, after the nonedible portions of the sugar cane or sugar beet have been removed.

regulated additive A food additive that has potentially toxic effects but when used in regulated amounts may be beneficial. A tolerance level is established for the use of the regulated additive, based on results of tests on laboratory animals. The U.S. Food and Drug Administration usually establishes a level for use of the additive in foods for human consumption.

rennin An enzyme that coagulates, or curdles, milk to make it easier for other digestive juices to break down. Rennin occurs naturally in the stomachs of human infants before they develop the pepsin enzyme. Rennin also occurs in the stomachs of calves and is utilized as a therapeutic digestive enzyme, and a dried extract, called *rennet*, is used in the manufacture of cheese and junkets or custards. Also called *chymosin; rennase*.

resistance training A type of fitness exercise program that involves working various muscle groups against some forms of resistance. Resistance training may employ the use of weights, dumbbells, or the counterforce of one's own body or that of a partner, making deliberately slow movements with muscular tensions and countertensions. See *weight lifting*.

restoration The replacement of vitamins and minerals in food products for those lost in milling and processing, with minimum and maximum levels specified. See *enriched cereal products; enrichment standards*.

retinal The name of a substance with vitamin A activity that is involved in the functions of vision, particularly color vision. Retinal combines with chemicals called *opsins* that are present in the cone cells of the retina, the light-sensitive surface on the inside of the eyeball, to form the pigments for the primary colors of vision. Retinal is a variation of vitamin A-1, which is also known as *retinol*. See *vitamin A*.

retinol See *vitamin A*.

rhodopsin See *visual purple*.

riboflavin A B-complex vitamin, also known as vitamin B-2, that appears as a yellow crystalline powder when isolated or synthesized and is involved in the metabolic processes of all living cells. Symptoms of riboflavin deficiency include a general weakness, loss of weight, redness and soreness of the tongue, lesions at the corners of the mouth and on the lips and nose, and a type of skin rash involving the oil glands. This vitamin deficiency also results in visual effects, particularly changes in the cornea.

Riboflavin had been known for many years, not as a vitamin but rather as a yellowish or greenish fluorescent substance in foods. The word *flavin* is derived from Latin and indicates something that is yellow in color. So the riboflavin in eggs was called *ovoflavin*, the riboflavin in milk was *lactoflavin*, the riboflavin in liver was *hepatoflavin*, and so on. But it was not realized at first that all the different flavins were the same substance. Scientists were aware, however, that when laboratory animals were given a diet rich in ovoflavin they grew faster. Other scientists in the early years of the twentieth century were aware that there was a growth-promoting substance in cereal grains besides the antiberiberi factor, now known as thiamine. When the outer coatings of grains are cooked at temperatures that destroy thiamine, there still remains a growth factor. The factor was temporarily given the name of vitamin G, for growth, by American researchers.

Around 1935, all the pieces began to fall into place. The various flavins, vitamin G, and a substance sometimes called the *yellow enzyme* turned out to be the same thing, a chemical the British had dubbed vitamin B-2, for the second of the water-soluble B factors in cereals, yeast, and liver. The enzyme relationship was cleared up when scientists realized that the substance was a coenzyme, the first of the vitamins to be shown to have such a metabolic function. In renaming the vitamin, the scientists agreed to keep the "flavin" part of the term but decided to add to the front of the name the word-fragment *ribo* because the molecular structure contained a chain of atoms resembling that of a sugar known as ribose.

As noted previously, riboflavin is more resistant to heat than thiamine. But it is almost as sensitive to light as photographic film. In fact, some studies of riboflavin must be carried out in a darkened laboratory because a flash of light on a sample of pure riboflavin could destroy it. Riboflavin is also sensitive to ultraviolet light, which is invisible to humans. However, it is only slightly soluble in water so little of the vitamin is lost in cooking.

The best sources of riboflavin are organ meats, such as liver and kidney, liver sausage, cheese, eggs, milk, and green leafy vegetables, plus whole grains and legumes. Sprouting seeds contain more riboflavin than other grains and younger plant materials are richer in riboflavin than older plant parts. A deficiency of riboflavin is more difficult to demonstrate in humans than some of the other nutrients and deficiency signs may take several months appear. To produce deficiency symptoms in less than a month, researchers have had to resort to the use of riboflavin antagonists. Even then, not all of the volunteer subjects showed precisely the same pattern of symptoms.

As thiamine becomes involved in metabolic processes leading to the formation of carbon dioxide, riboflavin functions as a coenzyme in metabolic activities in which hydrogen is passed along from one substance to another and finally converted to water to be excreted. By passing along hydrogen atoms, riboflavin helps break down carbohydrates, fatty acids, and amino acids, releasing energy to the tissue cells with each step of the process.

Also, like thiamine, the amount of riboflavin required by an individual is linked to the amount of calories burned during daily activities. The nutritional rule-of-thumb for riboflavin requirements is that one needs about 3/10 of 1 mg. of the vitamin for each 1,000 calories of energy burned. That proportion works out to around 1 mg. of riboflavin per day for small children, who may burn about 1,600 calories daily, to 2 mg. for a teenage boy who probably uses around 3,500 calories daily. Pregnant and nursing women need more than the usual amounts estimated for adult women. Also called *vitamin B-2; vitamin G.*

ribonucleic acid   A chemical that occurs naturally in all living cells and is responsible for the manufacture of protein molecules. Ribonucleic acid (RNA) is similar to deoxyribonucleic acid (DNA) and can replace DNA in certain situations. There are several kinds of ribonucleic acid. One kind, *messenger RNA*, carries the genetic code from the DNA in the nucleus of the cell to the cytoplasm. *Transfer RNA* transfers specific amino acid molecules to proteins being formed; there is a different transfer RNA for each amino acid. *Ribosomal RNA* is found in ribosomes, particles inside the cells that are also concerned with protein synthesis. Abbreviated *RNA.*

rice diet   A diet consisting mainly of rice, with sugar and fruit, introduced in the 1940s for people suffering from hypertension and kidney disease. The original version of the rice diet restricted the use of milk, fat, and sodium and provided about 2,000 calories daily with virtually no sodium. A more recent modified

rickets

form of the rice diet, intended for weight loss, reduces the caloric level considerably while increasing sodium content about fourfold by adding nonfat milk or butter to the rice, sugar, and fruit. This diet is not recommended for general use because it is deficient in protein, iron, some B vitamins, and vitamin A.

rickets   A nutritional deficiency disease of infancy and childhood caused by a lack of vitamin D, which in turn results in abnormal calcium and phosphorus metabolism and poor bone development. Because of the relationship between sunlight and vitamin D, rickets tends to occur in regions where winters are long, where smoke or fog prevent sunlight from reaching the ground, and among dark-skinned people whose skin color blocks the sunlight. Symptoms include soft and irregular bones, with bowlegs, knock-knee, and misshapen skulls some common effects. This disease can be prevented with the help of vitamin D-fortified milk. See *osteomalacia*.

risk/benefit   A formula used by the U.S. Food and Drug Administration in determining the accepted use of additives in food products by weighing the risks against the benefits. One example is the use of nitrites in cured meats, a situation in which it is accepted that nitrites may be a source of nitrosamines that cause cancer in laboratory animals—the risk—but at the same time they have been used for many generations to protect meats against botulism and other forms of food poisoning—the benefit. Because the chance of food poisoning without nitrites is greater than the risk of stomach cancer from using nitrites, the additive has been accepted.

roughage   See *fiber; bulk*.

rubidium   A chemical element that is a trace mineral found in the tissues of normal, healthy humans. Whether the mineral is essential is controversial. Rubidium has been used in medications, particularly for the treatment of nervous and mental disorders, but there is a lack of evidence that a deficiency of rubidium causes adverse health effects. The average North American diet contains adequate amounts of rubidium. This mineral functions in many ways like potassium and has been used experimentally to replace potassium in the bodies of small laboratory animals without ill effects. However, the same results would not occur in humans.

rutin   See *bioflavonoids*.

S

salt substitutes Chemical compounds that are available for flavoring food without adding sodium to the diet. Among substitutes for common table salt, which is sodium chloride, are potassium chloride, monopotassium glutamate, and glutamic acid. One or more brands of a mixture of sodium chloride and potassium chloride—to reduce the sodium proportion—may be available at one's grocery or drugstore. Salts that are identified as garlic salt or onion salt are not true salt substitutes because they are merely sodium chloride preparations with flavoring. See *potassium chloride*.

satiety center A region in the hypothalamus part of the brain that signals the rest of the body that eating should stop after a satisfactory amount of food has entered the stomach. The satiety center is needed to prevent overeating. It is believed that this center is able to detect changes in blood sugar levels after a meal is underway and sends out a stop-eating signal when the level reaches a certain high point in the blood. In experimental animals, damage to the hypothalamus results in the animals eating continuously regardless of the need for food.

satiety value The capacity of a food to sustain the sense of fullness, and to prevent an early renewal of hunger. Fat, for example, slows up the rate of digestion which contributes to a delay in the urge to eat.

saturated fat A food fat composed of saturated fatty acids, or fatty acids with molecules that are saturated with hydrogen molecules. A saturated fat is generally a solid fat because adding hydrogen atoms to a fatty acid makes it more solid and less liquid, if it was previously unsaturated. As a rule-of-thumb, a fat that is solid at room temperature is a saturated fat. Butter, margarine, and most animal fats contain saturated fatty acids.

scratch test A method of testing the reaction of a person to a possible allergen by scratching the skin on the arm or back and placing small samples of suspected allergens in the scratch marks. If the patient is allergic to a substance, a rash or other skin eruption will appear in the scratch.

scurvy A disease caused by a lack of vitamin C, or ascorbic acid, and marked by tissue degeneration disorders, such as loose teeth, bleeding and swollen gums, rupture of small blood vessels, small bruises of the skin, anemia, weakness, and soreness of the arms and legs. In advanced cases, there may also be heart and breathing irregularities. Scurvy in infants may also produce symptoms of irritability, poor appetite, digestive problems, and failure to gain weight. These disorders respond rapidly to vitamin C in the diet. The term scurvy is derived from an old Scandinavian word *scurf,* meaning "scars or scabs." See *vitamin C.*

second wind See *oxygen debt.*

selenium A mineral found in small amounts in the human body where it serves as a cofactor of an enzyme involved in maintaining membrane structures. It is also incorporated into muscle enzymes and in myoglobin, a form of hemoglobin that occurs in muscle tissues. Selenium can substitute for sulfur in some amino acid structures and reactions, but sulfur does not substitute for selenium in its roles. Selenium occurs in the body in amounts of 2 parts per 10-million. The amounts in food sources vary locally because of differences of the mineral in the soil; however, this seldom affects humans, who eat a wide variety of foods from a number of geographic areas.

sequestrant A substance that combines with metals to form complexes that are no longer able to become involved in chemical reactions. As used in foods, sequestrants deactivate metals that otherwise would increase the rate of oxidation and spoilage of the food. The overall effect is to prevent the food from becoming rancid and losing its original color, flavor, and odor. Sequestrants protect the potency of vitamins in a similar manner. They are commonly used to protect fish, meat, and dairy products. Some sequestrants, such as citric and tartaric acid, provide additional benefits by changing the acidity of the food.

serine A nonessential amino acid present in many types of animal proteins, including casein, egg albumin, and collagen. It is used by the body in forming the fibrin of blood clots and in such enzymes and hormones as pepsin and insulin.

serotonin A powerful neurotransmitter derived with the help of enzymes from the amino acid tryptophan. Serotonin is involved primarily in helping nerve impulses across synapses in the brain cells. It is particularly concerned with nerve messages related to wakefulness, temperature of the body, and blood pressure regulation. Monoamine oxidase is one of the possible metabolic by-products of the breakdown of serotonin molecules. A substance found in the digestive tract, enteramine, is a close chemical relative of serotonin.

side effects Effects of a drug or nutrient that are in addition to the intended effect. The side effect of penicillin in a sensitive person, for example, may be a severe skin rash, whereas symptoms of purpura may be side effects of aspirin or acetaminophen. Also called *adverse reactions*. See *food-drug interaction; hypervitaminosis*.

silicon A trace mineral found in human skin and connective tissues. Diseases of the connective tissues are sometimes associated with a deficiency of silicon in the body. The required amount in the human body is not known at this time; in experiments, the amount excreted equals the amount ingested, suggesting that the body maintains a constant level. Silicon is found in certain molecules of the body chemistry that are complexes of sugars and amino acids. In nature's food sources, silicon occurs in unpolished rice and certain cereals, particularly those used in making beer.

single-cell protein A term sometimes used to identify food yeasts that are produced as a rich source of protein. Food yeasts are approximately one-third protein and contain as many as 18 of the 22 known amino acids. Abbreviated *SCP*.

Sippy diet A diet developed by American physician Bertram Sippy for people who are unable to consume bulky foods because of peptic ulcers or other digestive disorders. The diet is limited to milk and cream for the first few days, but other foods, such as crackers, cereals, eggs, and puréed vegetables are gradually added to the diet so that by the end of the month the patient is usually able to eat regular foods with the exception of items that might aggravate the condition, such as chili con carne.

skinfold thickness The measurement, with an instrument called a *caliper*, of the thickness of a pinch of skin at a selected place such as the upper arm, or just below the shoulder blade or upper abdomen. These measurements indicate the amount of fat beneath the skin, which tells the state of the body's nutrition.

small calorie An alternate term for *gram calorie*, or the amount of heat required to raise the temperature of 1 g. of water by 1°C. See *calorie; gram calorie; kilocalorie*.

smooth diet A diet for people with peptic ulcers. It is similar to the Sippy diet, with little or no roughage. Coarse breads or cereals and raw fruits and vegetables are usually excluded. Farina and applesauce might be acceptable but shredded wheat and raw apples would be prohibited.

soda water A mixture of water and carbon dioxide. Because the carbonated beverage was made from sodium salts, like sodium bicarbonate, when invented in the eighteenth century, the word "soda" has been associated with the beverage although sodium salts are no longer used. Modern soda water is manufactured simply by injecting pure carbon dioxide gas into pure water. Soda water may be the only soft drink that contains no additives, colorings, flavorings, or sweeteners. Also called *club soda.*

sodium A mineral found in relatively large amounts in the body's fluids and which has a primary function of maintaining fluid pressure and balance. The body contains an average of approximately 3 oz. of sodium, most of it dissolved in the extracellular fluids—or fluids outside the body cells—and in the blood. In the dissolved state, sodium occurs as a positively charged ion, or a more or less free-floating atom carrying a positive electrical charge. Such an ion is also known as an electrolyte.

The sodium ions and those of potassium and other dissolved elements regulate the acid-base balance of the blood and other body tissues, control the excretion of sodium and potassium in the urine, and influence the functions of nerves and muscle fibers. The electrical charges on sodium ions outside a nerve cell and those on potassium ions inside the cell provide the electrical energy for transmission of a nerve impulse along a fiber extension of the cell. The movement of sodium and potassium ions across the nerve membrane, a process called a *sodium pump,* accounts in part for changes in the electrical charge of a nerve cell.

Irregularities in sodium levels in the body are associated with behavioral changes; an increase in sodium levels accompanies an episode of depression and a group of symptoms called a low-sodium syndrome is marked by psychotic behavior. An excess of sodium in the blood has profound effects on the central nervous system, with confusion, stupor, and coma. Psychiatrists believe these effects are caused by dehydration of the brain cells by the excess sodium. Sodium depletion causes nausea, vomiting, signs of shock, and a condition called *water intoxication,* in which ordinary water produces effects similar to those caused by drinking whiskey or another alcoholic beverage. Water intoxication is representative of the condition resulting from an electrolyte imbalance in the body tissues. In addition to psychiatric symptoms created by a sodium imbalance, increasing the sodium intake of the body results in an equivalent increase in fluid retention; hormonal regulators attempt to ensure that proportions of water to sodium in the body are constant. Increased fluid retention accounts for several serious disorders ranging from high blood pressure to premenstrual tension.

Major sources of sodium in the diet are ordinary table salt, or sodium chloride, and additives like monosodium glutamate (MSG). Salt in various forms is added liberally to food during processing because it retards the growth of microorganisms, most of which need water to survive; salt deprives them of the water in the food. Preserved meats, such as pork products, salted nuts and crackers, ketchup, mustard, brined pickles, olives, and many canned foods, contain added salts. Bakery products contain sodium from the use of sodium bicarbonate in their processing. Thus, sodium deficiencies seldom occur in people who eat a typical modern diet of processed foods. However, vegetables before processing are not a rich source of sodium and vegans, or pure vegetarians, who prepare their meals from fresh raw fruits and vegetables may find it necessary to add some table salt. Most adults can live normal, healthy lives with no more than 4 or 5 g. of sodium each day to replace losses through perspiration and excretion. People who sweat a lot from hard work or exercise often require larger doses, and salt may be recommended during illness to replace losses from vomiting or diarrhea. See *low sodium diet*.

sodium benzoate A food additive used as a preservative in margarines, fruit juices, pickles, and other products. It is one of several food substances that tastes differently to different individuals. Sodium benzoate is commonly added to non–heat-treated soft drinks because it increases the acidity of the beverage to a level that retards spoilage by bacteria. Also called *benzoate of soda*.

sodium bicarbonate See *bicarbonate of soda*.

sodium chloride See *table salt*.

soft diet A diet that consists mainly of soft foods, such as eggs, milk, ice cream, custards, tapioca or rice puddings, applesauce, fruit juices, mashed potatoes, and other foods that require little or no chewing and a minimum of roughage. Soft diets are sometimes recommended for people who have no teeth, as well as for those with gastrointestinal disorders.

soft drinks A common name for carbonated nonalcoholic beverages. Soft drinks are generally composed of water, sugar, flavorings, colorings, acids, and carbon dioxide. The original soft drinks were created in ancient Greek and Roman days, using naturally occurring mineral waters, and consumed for their reputed medicinal benefits. In 1767, British scientist Joseph Priestley discovered a method of making carbonated water artificially from sodium bicarbonate. Also called *soda; soda pop.* See *brominated vegetable oil; soda water*.

soft water A term used to identify water that contains less than 1 grain of calcium or magnesium mineral salts per gallon of water. There are 437 grains per ounce. Technically, soft water is defined as water that is so free of minerals that soap curd will not form in it. Government and other official agencies often classify water as soft when it contains less than 3 to 5 grains of mineral salts per gallon. Softened water is generally not regarded as being as healthful as hard water because hard water contains important minerals; artificially softened water may contain high levels of sodium, which is added to displace the calcium.

sorbitol   A sweet-tasting powder that is technically a type of alcohol but which is used as a sugar substitute that can be consumed by diabetes mellitus patients because it does not require normal insulin function to be metabolized. Sorbitol occurs naturally in fruits, such as apples, cherries, pears, peaches, and prunes. It is also found in red seaweed. Sorbitol is used commercially in mouth washes and toothpastes because it resists the microbial activity associated with tooth decay from sugar in the mouth. Sorbitol is converted to fructose in the liver and can be produced synthetically from glucose molecules.

spring water   Water that flows naturally from an underground spring and is not obtained by the use of electric or other pumping devices. Spring water, like artesian water, is rich in minerals as a result of flowing over rock layers of the earth. The water is generally the runoff of rainfall that has seeped undergound and followed rocky pathways to an opening in the surface. See *mineral water*.

sprue   See *celiac-sprue; tropical sprue*.

staminal principles   A term introduced in the nineteenth century when it was believed that an adequate diet consisted of fats, carbohydrates, and proteins, which were identified as the three staminal principles needed for a healthy life. Staminal was derived from the Latin word *stamen*, for "thread of life."

standards of identity   See *food standards of identity*.

St. Anthony's fire   A common name for *ergotism*, a disease caused by eating cereal grains contaminated by ergot fungus. Symptoms include a dry gangrene of the extremities, convulsions, and painful muscular contractions. This disease was common in the Middle Ages, and as recently as the eighteenth century, because moldy grain was used in making bread. An Italian monastery named for St. Anthony provided victims with bread that was free of ergot and became a refuge where patients could recover—even though neither the monks nor the victims understood at the time that it was ergot-free bread rather than the pilgrimage to St. Anthony's shrine that accounted for relief from the disease symptoms.

starch   A white, tasteless, odorless powder or mass of fine granules composed of hundreds to thousands of glucose molecules linked together by chemical bonds. When subjected to heat and water, the granules split into layers and form a paste. When subjected to dry heat, starch is converted to *dextrin*, also called *starch gum*, which is further reduced to glucose units in the presence of water. Digestive enzymes break down starch into units of glucose, maltose, and dextrin. See *carbohydrates*.

steatorrhea The term for a condition in which excess fat appears in the feces. The cause is generally a malabsorption syndrome related to a disease involving the lining of the intestinal tract or a deficiency of the pancreatic enzymes or liver bile needed to metabolize fats. Steatorrhea may also result from severe malnutrition. Normally, about 95 percent of fats in the diet are absorbed and very little is excreted. See *idiopathic steatorrhea*.

sterols The name of a group of organic chemical compounds that have characteristics of both fats and alcohol. One example is cholesterol. Another example is ergosterol, a substance in ergot and yeast that is converted to vitamin D-2, or calciferol, when it is irradiated with ultraviolet light.

strontium A chemical element found in human body tissues in trace amounts. The role of strontium in human nutrition is not fully understood. It competes with calcium for absorption and is usually excreted before calcium; strontium also follows the same pathways as calcium through the body. Most of the strontium in the body is concentrated in the bones. One study showed that strontium may be necessary for calcium to be deposited properly in teeth and bones, but some authorities have challenged that claim. A radioactive isotope, strontium-90, may enter the body from fallout of nuclear explosions.

subclinical deficiency The deficiency of a nutrient that is so small it does not produce any serious health signs or symptoms, even though laboratory tests show below normal levels in the body. One example is the slow healing of a wound that may be caused by a deficiency of zinc or of vitamin C, which could be detected by careful laboratory tests but would likely be ignored by the patient unless the wound interfered with work, play, or social life.

sucrose A form of sugar that consists of two simple sugars, fructose and glucose, linked by a chemical bond. It is the most widely distributed of the various forms of sugar, occurring in ripe fruits, sugar beets, and sugar cane. Table sugar, or granulated sugar, is a commercial form of sucrose. It is also used in manufacturing caramel since it loses water and forms a brown syrup when heated.

sugar The term applied to any sweet-tasting carbohydrate that may be found in plant or animal tissues. Sugars are usually classified according to the number of basic carbohydrate units in their molecules. A monosaccharide, for example, is a simple, basic sugar molecule, whereas a disaccharide contains two of the basic sugar units. Large complexes of sugar units become starch or cellulose. Ordinary table sugar is a disaccharide, sucrose, composed of one unit of glucose and one of fructose, that has been refined. Natural unrefined sugar is brown because it has not been bleached. See *cellulose; starch*.

sugar alcohol   A sweet-tasting alcohol that occurs naturally in various fruits and appears as a white powder when extracted. Examples of sugar alcohols include *mannitol* and *sorbitol*. See these entries.

sulfur   A chemical element and essential mineral in human nutrition. Four of the amino acids—cysteine, cystine, methionine, and taurine—require sulfur atoms in their structures. If the diet includes enough methionine, the other amino acids can be synthesized with the sulfur in the essential amino acid. Sulfur compounds are found in the saliva, bile, blood corpuscles, and the processes of oxidation in the tissue cells. The body requires approximately 1 g. of sulfur per day in food items. Sulfur supplements are rarely if ever needed.

supplement   Any vitamin or other nutrient consumed in addition to nutrients in the foods eaten.

sweet almond   A relative of the bitter almond, but with a kernel that lacks the toxic cyanide compound of bitter almonds. The sweet almond, which also grows in the Mediterranean area, has been used as a food source since Biblical times. It can be eaten as a raw nut, slivered, ground, fried, baked, or made into a paste. Sweet almonds contain about as much protein per ounce as beef, plus linoleic acid, thiamine, riboflavin, niacin, iron, calcium, potassium, and phosphorus.

symptom   Any health abnormality that is perceived by the person affected, as distinguished from *signs*, which are health effects observed by doctors or other persons. Some physical complaints, such as a toothache or a feeling of fatigue, are symptoms because another person would not be able to perceive the same feelings, although that person might be able to detect signs of pain or fatigue from the behavior of the patient.

syndrome   A combination of several symptoms or signs of ill health that are related to a single cause. Syndromes are usually identified according to their specific causes, effects, or the name of the doctor who first described the condition. One example is a condition known as the *stiff-man syndrome*, which is characterized by overdeveloped muscles, painful muscle spasms, and clubfoot or a similar foot deformity, all related to a problem of phosphorus metabolism.

synthesis   The process whereby something is created or manufactured from other materials. In the human body, nonessential amino acids can be synthesized from essential amino acids that contribute the necessary materials. Synthesis may also refer to the commercial processes of manufacturing food or other products from organic or inorganic materials. See *synthetic food colors; synthetic food flavors; synthetic vitamins.*

synthetic food colors Food colors that are manufactured from coal tar or other sources. Food colors that are listed as FD&C (for food, drugs and cosmetics) followed by a number are synthetic colors. Food processors often used synthetic colors where natural colors are not stable or otherwise satisfactory for foods that may have to be on a supermarket shelf for weeks or months after cooking and canning. For example, FD&C Red No. 40 may be used to color candy, soft drinks, maraschino cherries, bakery products, and other items because a natural food color like beet juice would deteriorate, interact with enzymes in the foods, or otherwise produce off-colors and off-flavors.

synthetic food flavors Chemical compounds that are used alone or in blends or combinations to produce a flavor that resembles a natural fruit or vegetable taste in a food or beverage. More than 1,000 synthetic flavors are used in various processed foods. One example of a synthetic food flavor is linalyl benzoate, a chemical that is used to create peach, citrus, and berry flavors in beverages, ice cream, gelatin desserts, candy, and bakery products. One of the synthetic raspberry flavors contains 29 different chemicals, ranging from 2 parts biacetyl to 400 parts ethylmethylphenylglycidate.

synthetic vitamins Vitamins that are manufactured from chemical components, as distinguished from natural vitamins that are extracted from foods which are rich sources of these vitamins. There is essentially no difference between synthetic and natural vitamins, but natural vitamins are generally more expensive because of the difficulty of extracting them from fish oils or other sources. Vitamins used in vitamin supplements are usually the most stable form of the nutrient because of the need to retard deterioration and handling effects.

systolic A term commonly applied to the blood pressure reading that reflects the pressure of the heart contraction. Blood pressure readings measure the pressure of the blood being forced through the arteries and against the resistance of arterial walls and other factors. The pressure is usually at a high point immediately after a systole, or contraction of the lower heart chambers, and at a low point when the heart is in one of its brief moments of relaxation between contractions. The blood pressure during the heart's relaxation phase is called *diastolic.* Blood pressure readings are written as systolic/diastolic and may appear as 120/80, the numbers indicating millimeters of mercury. The numbers indicate the patient's systolic blood pressure has enough force to raise a column of mercury in a glass tube a distance of 120 millimeters. See *blood pressure; diastolic.*

t

table salt The common name of sodium chloride, a compound of 1 part sodium to 1 part chlorine. The average daily intake of table salt by North Americans is between ¼ and ½ of 1 oz., which provides between 3 to 6 g. of sodium. People on low-sodium diets, which limit daily intake to between 250 and 1,000 mg. of sodium per day, can usually get along without table salt because natural or processed foods provide that much sodium in the diet. Also called *sodium chloride*. See *iodized salt*.

tablet The form in which dried and granulated or powdered drugs are compressed and molded. A tablet is usually round but may be molded into an oval or other shape. They contain a binder of casein or starch that disintegrates in water to disperse the other substances. Some tablets use moistened sugar as a binder. Some are scored so they can be broken into halves or quarters. Tablets may also be engraved or marked with an initial or symbol that identifies the contents or the manufacturer.

temperature regulation The process of maintaining a constant body temperature through metabolic heat production or by mechanisms that eliminate excessive body heat. When the temperature of the environment is too high, the body's arteries near the surface of the skin dilate so that heat can be dissipated through the skin. About 70 percent of excess body heat is dissipated in this manner. An additional 25 percent is dissipated through the evaporation of moisture from the surface of the skin, or sweating. Between 1 and 2 percent is lost through excretion. Only 3 percent is used to compensate for the lower temperature of air, foods, and beverages, brought into the body.

tetany A continuous muscle spasm or contraction that may occur without significant signs of twitching. However, in some cases tetany may be accompanied by cramps, convulsions, and sharp muscle flexions. The cause is a deficiency of calcium in the blood that results in irritability of the nerves and muscles. Tetany may be associated with an inadequate intake of calcium or vitamin D, the loss of parathyroid glands, or underactive parathyroid glands. Tetany can also result from alkalosis, particularly when vomiting causes a serious loss of electrolytes.

theobromine A substance obtained from cocoa that is similar to caffeine in its effects on the body. Theobromine affects all the body systems influenced by caffeine and theophylline but is less potent than either of its chemical cousins. See *caffeine; theophylline.*

theophylline A substance that is closely related to caffeine and is present in tea leaves. Theophylline has effects on the body's physiology that are similar to those of caffeine but in a different degree. For example, caffeine is more potent as a central nervous system and respiratory stimulant, but theophylline is more potent as a heart stimulant, as a diuretic, and as a smooth muscle relaxant.

therapeutic A term that refers to the cure or treatment of a disease or injury. The term is derived from an ancient Greek word *therapeia,* meaning "service to the sick."

therapeutic diet A term applied to a diet prescribed by a doctor, to be used as part of a treatment program that also includes medication, an exercise plan, or other nondietary procedures. One example is a diet for diabetes mellitus patients that is designed to combine the use of a certain daily dose of insulin and an exercise plan that balances daily caloric intake.

thiamine The first of the B vitamins to be discovered, hence its other name of vitamin B-1. Thiamine is important in carbohydrate metabolism and in all processes that eventually yield carbon dioxide as a waste product. The amount of thiamine required by an individual is so closely linked to carbohydrate metabolism that a person suffering from thiamine deficiency requires long periods of rest to conserve the thiamine in his tissues; physical activity that burns calories depletes the thiamine. Thiamine occurs naturally in nearly all plant and animal food sources, although some are much better sources than others.

The effects of thiamine deficiency were known for at least 50 years before the vitamin was discovered. Like vitamin C, the antiscurvy vitamin, thiamine research was given a boost by a health problem of sailors. The Japanese Navy sailed into the same ports of the Orient as the British Navy during the nineteenth century, but up to 40 percent of Japanese sailors were disabled at any time because of beriberi. Symptoms included heart and liver disorders, nervous irritability, debility and paralysis, excessive weight loss, and eventually death. Many doctors were convinced that beriberi was caused by an infectious microorganism, but one Japanese officer decided as an experiment to give the men aboard one ship the same kinds of foods eaten by the British sailors. Somewhat miraculously, most of the Japanese sailors in the experiment were not afflicted with beriberi. However, some sailors in the experiment still suffered from beriberi and it was feared the British diet would not be the answer; that is, until investigation showed that the sailors still plagued by beriberi were not following the British diet but had instead been preparing their own meals in the traditional manner with polished rice. When the convincing evidence of the diet was presented to the Japanese Admiralty, the food served Japanese sailors was changed and beriberi was eliminated within 2 years.

In another part of the Orient meanwhile, a team of scientists sent from The Netherlands to the Dutch East Indies to study beriberi decided to test the theory that the disease was caused by bacteria by injecting chickens with samples of blood taken from beriberi patients. When the chickens developed peculiar behavior patterns soon after, swaying about with wings drooping, the researchers believed they had proof that beriberi was an infectious disease. Then it was discovered that the chickens were being fed the leftovers of polished rice served persons with beriberi. But the link between the polished rice and beriberi was missed again. The chickens were returned to a diet of unpolished rice eaten by the natives because it was cheaper than the polished rice. Then the chickens recovered. Still the thiamine factor was missing and scientists turned their attention to viruses and fungi as possible beriberi causes.

Confounding the misinformation about beriberi was the unintentional introduction of the disease in the Philippine Islands after the Spanish-American War of 1898. Beriberi was virtually unknown in the Philippines until well-meaning Americans decided that as a matter of social welfare, prisoners should be fed polished rice instead of their native form of the cereal. Within the first year thousands of prisoners were afflicted with beriberi and hundreds died. As the use of polished rice spread to the civil population, deaths from beriberi in the Philippines rose to nearly 25,000 per year, even after the substance now called thiamine was isolated from rice polishings in Indonesia in 1926. Another decade passed before thiamine could be analyzed and synthesized. Then it was given its name, derived from *thio*, meaning "sulfur-containing," and *amine*, because it contains an amino chemical group. It was the first vitamin ever obtained from food in pure form.

After knowledge of the role of thiamine was established, a group of scientists conducted an experiment in which subjects volunteered to live on a diet that included thiamine, but in amounts less than normal. Within 10 days, the volunteers became depressed, irritable, and unable to concentrate. In 3 weeks, they began to experience fatigue, loss of appetite and body weight, constipation, and muscle cramps. When the thiamine content of their food was increased, they quickly regained normal health. Although thiamine is present in almost all natural foods, few foods are rich sources of thiamine. The best sources are whole grains, legumes, pork, and organ meats. What is available in the thiamine content of common foods is often reduced or destroyed by cooking because thiamine is very heat sensitive. Large amounts of live yeast in the diet can block the absorption of thiamine from the intestinal tract. Raw fish and other seafood, such as shrimp and clams, contain an enzyme called *thiaminase* which destroys thiamine. Because thiamine is highly soluble in water, the vitamin can be lost in cooking water, unless the water is also used as part of the meal. Also called *vitamin B-1; antiberiberi factor.*

thiamine deficiency See *athiaminosis.*

threonine An essential amino acid important for growth and nitrogen equilibrium in humans. Threonine is considered a glucogenic amino acid because it is metabolized into substances that are easily converted to glucose.

thrombin An enzyme that is important to the blood-clotting process because of its ability to convert fibrinogen into fibrin, the meshlike network of fibers that is the foundation of the clot.

thrombosis The presence or formation of a blood clot, or *thrombus*, inside a blood vessel or in one of the heart chambers. A thrombus can block or retard the normal flow of blood through an artery or vein, causing a stroke, heart attack, or other health emergency. Thrombosis is usually identified by its location, such as *coronary thrombosis*, if in a coronary artery of the heart; *arterial thrombosis*, if in an artery; or *venous thrombosis*, if located in a vein.

thyroid hormones The hormones produced by the thyroid gland, which is located in the neck. They include thyroxine and triiodothyronine, which stimulate specific organs and tissue cells of the body, controlling such factors as a person's skeletal growth, level of energy, sexual development, skin texture, and hair luster. A third thyroid hormone, calcitonin, influences the levels of calcium and phosphorus in the blood and absorption of the minerals by the bones.

timed release A term applied to tablets or capsules that deliver their ingredients in small, gradual amounts over a period of several hours. Some vitamins are manufactured in timed-release formulations but so many factors influence the effectiveness of the method, such as individual differences in the amount of time it takes substances to travel through the digestive tract, that the need for timed-release vitamins has been questioned by authorities.

tin A nutrient that occurs naturally in many foods and in body tissues. The distribution of tin in human body tissues has been calculated to average about 2 parts per 10-million. Frozen, fresh, and bottled foods generally contain less than 2 µg. of tin. But food samples from unlacquered food cans may contain more than 50 µg. of tin, and food stored in open unlacquered cans in a refrigerator can contribute excessive amounts of tin to the human diet.

It is estimated that about 15 percent of Americans commonly consume food from an open can stored in a refrigerator. A person who consumes ½ lb. of food from an opened unlacquered can stored in a refrigerator, according to nutrition scientists, may have a daily intake of as much as 100 mg. of tin, which is several thousand times the amount of tin one might consume in fresh, frozen, or bottled foods.

The effects of small amounts of tin on human health are inconclusive. A study of men who consumed diets containing tin in the amounts found in open unlacquered cans stored in refrigerators showed abnormal zinc metabolism, with less zinc retained from foods eaten, and possible changes in their copper metabolism. Other studies of laboratory animals found growth was retarded from both too much and too little tin in the diet. Tin appears to be involved in the formation of proteins and in certain enzyme functions. It is classified as a microelement, meaning only very tiny amounts of this mineral are required in the daily diet.

tocopherol The name of a group of substances that are technically alcohols and have vitamin E activity. Tocopherol can be manufactured synthetically or obtained from food sources, such as wheat germ and other grains, vegetables, and fruits. After wheat-germ oil, the cereal seed oils—soybean, cottonseed, and corn—are the richest sources of tocopherols. Milk and potatoes are among the poorest food sources. Of the four major types of tocopherol, alpha-tocopherol is the most potent. The others are identified as beta-, gamma-, and delta-tocopherol. See *alpha-tocopherol; vitamin E.*

tongue tie See *ankylglossia.*

torutilin The name of a substance obtained from torula yeast and sometimes identified as vitamin T because of its ability to produce abnormally rapid growth in insects. It is claimed that torutilin is able to stimulate rapid growth and regeneration of diseased or injured human tissues.

toxicity The quality of being poisonous, usually expressed as a degree of danger to life or health. Anything in the environment, including oxygen, water, and sunlight, can be toxic, or poisonous, when used in excess of normal amounts. The exact amount of any substance that may be toxic to any individual is not possible to predict accurately, but toxic levels of most chemicals have been estimated on the basis of animal experiments. Experimental results are recorded as the *minimum lethal dose*, the smallest amount of the substance needed to kill an animal, or the amount required to kill half the animals. The dangerous dose for humans is extrapolated from the lethal dose for experimental animals.

toxoplasmosis A disease caused by protozoa, one-celled microorganisms, causing symptoms that may resemble those of infectious mononucleosis or more serious effects, including damage to the heart, lungs, brain, liver, skin, and muscle. Toxoplasmosis can be acquired by humans from eating meat that has not been properly cooked. When a pregnant woman is infected, the protozoa can cross the placental barrier and infect the fetus, causing blindness, brain defects, or death. The National Livestock and Meat Board recommends that all meat be heated to at least 140°F (60°C), the "rare" reading on a meat thermometer, because many domestic animals are infected.

trace minerals Minerals required by the human body mainly as cofactors for metabolic functions in daily amounts of less than 1/2,000 of 1 oz. Also called *trace elements*.

transamination The process whereby the body's chemical mechanisms transfer an amino group, the nitrogen-containing portion of an amino acid, from one amino acid to another. By the transamination process, nonessential amino acids can be manufactured by the body from essential amino acids in the diet. Removal of the amino group is the first step in the metabolism of amino acids. If the amino group is not used to build another amino acid, it is usually converted to urea to be excreted.

transketolase An enzyme that converts chemicals from ketone bodies into pentose, a sugar molecule. Ketone bodies are derived in turn from fatty acids. Thiamine is a coenzyme of transketolase, and the metabolic step, which is important for certain blood cell functions, may not occur if there is a thiamine deficiency.

tranquilizers A group of drugs used to calm an agitated or anxious person without producing the effects of drowsiness associated with sedatives; some drowsiness may occur but the patient is easily aroused if necessary. Tranquilizers are usually divided into two groups: *minor tranquilizers*, or *antianxiety drugs*, prescribed mainly for people with excessive anxiety and tension; and *major tranquilizers*, or *neuroleptics*, prescribed for psychotically agitated people, those diagnosed as schizophrenic or in a manic-depressive state.

triceps A muscle that extends from the humerus, the upper arm bone, to the ulna, one of the two bones of the lower arm. The job of the triceps is to straighten the elbow joint. It works in tandem with the biceps, which bends the elbow joint. See *biceps*.

triglycerides Compounds composed of three molecules of fatty acids attached to a molecule of glycerin. Triglycerides are the usual form in which fats are stored in animal tissues and the level of triglycerides circulating in the blood is a measure of the risk of disease of the heart and circulatory system.

tropical sprue A disease that is a variation of celiac-sprue and that mainly affects people who live in tropical regions, particularly southern Asia and the Caribbean. The symptoms are similar to those of celiac-sprue but wheat gluten does not seem to be a factor. However, the lining of the small intestine is affected so that nutrients like folic acid and vitamin B-12 are not absorbed. Steatorrhea is common. See *celiac-sprue*.

tryptophan One of the essential amino acids which, like most other amino acids, is necessary for normal growth and nitrogen balance. Tryptophan is unique in being an amino acid that is a precursor of a vitamin, niacin. Experiments indicate that it can be a source of glucose through metabolic processes. It is also a precursor of the neurotransmitter serotonin and a source of metabolic products involved in blood clotting and the constriction of blood vessels. Meat, milk, eggs, and some leafy vegetables are food sources of tryptophan.

turista A popular name that originated in Mexico for a type of diarrhea experienced by travelers. It can be caused by bacterial toxins or viruses. Symptoms are similar to those of "intestinal flu" and include nausea, vomiting, abdominal cramps, and borborygmi, in addition to diarrhea. Also called *Montezuma's revenge*.

tyramine A substance produced by the metabolism of the amino acid tyrosine. Tyramine is found in dead animal tissue, ripe cheese, alcoholic beverages, pickled herring, and other items. Tyramine is related in chemical structure to the neurotransmitters epinephrine and norepinephrine and has a similar effect. Tyramine is normally broken down by an enzyme called *monoamine oxidase*, but this does not happen when an individual uses a drug that is a monoamine oxidase inhibitor. As a result, a reaction occurs with a flooding of the body by norepinephrine and symptoms of severe hypertension. See *monoamine oxidase inhibitors*.

tyrosine A naturally occurring amino acid that can be manufactured in the body from an essential amino acid, phenylalanine. Tyrosine is an important factor in the formation of the neurotransmitter epinephrine, the skin pigment melanin, and the hormone thyroxine produced by the thyroid gland. Two vitamins, C and B-12, are involved in the metabolic breakdown of tyrosine. Several inborn errors of metabolism are caused by a lack of enzymes for the complete metabolism of phenylalanine and tyrosine. They are phenylketonuria (PKU), tyrosinosis, and alcaptonuria.

u

ubiquinone Any of a group of quinones, the name of substances derived from the quinic acid of fruits, that are similar to vitamin K-1 in molecular structure and function and serve in metabolic processes by carrying electrons from one chemical compound to another. Also called *coenzyme Q*.

ulcer Any defect in an organ or tissue surface caused by a sloughing-off of dead inflamed tissue, leaving a small depression or excavation. An ulcer can appear anywhere on a body surface but the term is usually applied to ulcers that appear in the digestive tract. Digestive tract ulcers are identified as peptic ulcers, caused by the erosion of surfaces lining the esophagus, stomach, or intestine, and are also given names that indicate their specific location, such as gastric ulcer, for a stomach ulcer.

ultraviolet light The light wavelengths that are beyond the violet end of the spectrum and are therefore invisible to humans. Ultraviolet wavelengths of light produce the tanning and burning effects of the skin and are also the source of energy for converting provitamin D in the skin into vitamin D, which can be absorbed by the body. Artificial sources of ultraviolet light are used commercially to produce vitamin D-fortified foods. In producing vitamin D-fortified milk, for example, an appropriate substance in the milk, such as a form of cholesterol, is converted to vitamin D by exposing the milk to ultraviolet light.

undernutrition Inadequate intake of one or more nutrients or calories. See *subclinical deficiency*.

United States Food and Drug Administration An agency of the U.S. Department of Health and Human Services that is assigned the responsibility of protecting the health of the consumer against unsafe and impure foods, drugs, cosmetics, and other potential hazards. The agency is divided into five bureaus that control biological products, drugs, foods, radiation hazards, and veterinary medicine. A sixth division is the National Center for Toxicological

Research, which studies the effects of toxic substances in the environment and establishes toxicity standards through animal experiments. Abbreviated *FDA*.

unsaturated fat A fatty substance that contains unsaturated fatty acids. Most liquid vegetable oils are unsaturated fats. See *unsaturated fatty acids.*

unsaturated fatty acids Any of the fatty acid molecules that have bonds, or links between atoms, that can hold additional atoms of hydrogen. Unsaturated fatty acids are more likely to become rancid when exposed to air because oxygen atoms in the air can break down the fatty acid molecules at the point where there are no hydrogen molecules, turning them rancid. However, unsaturated fatty acids are generally easier to digest because they are liquids and they are also less likely to be involved in atherosclerosis, the degenerative disease of the arteries caused by eating excessive amounts of fatty foods.

urea A substance produced in the liver from amino acids and compounds containing ammonia. It is found in the blood, lymph, and urine. The amount of urea in the body increases with the amount of protein in the diet as the chemical mechanisms of the body remove the amino portions of amino acids absorbed from the intestinal tract. A significant amount of urea production is also associated with the normal wear-and-tear of body proteins, which are also stripped of their amino groups.

uremia A disorder caused by the accumulation in the blood of metabolic waste products that would normally be excreted by the kidneys. The failure of the kidneys to function properly may be caused in turn by an obstruction, disease, injury, or poisoning. Potassium and amino acid waste products are the primary substances that accumulate and cause symptoms of severe muscle weakness, a tingling of the facial muscles in the area of the mouth, and heart problems that may be fatal. Protein intake is usually restricted and dialysis is used to help remove excess potassium and other waste products.

uric acid An acid formed by the metabolism in the body of purine substances in foods. Purines are found mainly in animal food products, such as anchovies, sardines, and organ meats that include sweetbreads, kidney, and liver. An excess of uric acid in the body can be a cause of gout.

urine test The laboratory examination of a sample of urine to determine signs of an abnormality in a metabolic or kidney function. The examination may include an inspection for color and odor, a microscopic study of red and white blood cells that may be present, a check for the presence of crystals or mineral deposits, pus or bacteria, and chemical tests for glucose, albumin, and other substances. There are a number of different urine tests, including a diaper test for phenylketonuria in infants, urea nitrogen (BUN), and urinary flow rate.

uroflavin The name of a compound found in the urine and closely related to riboflavin. It appears in urine samples following an intake of riboflavin.

urticaria A medical term used to identify a kind of skin disorder marked by swelling in small areas or small raised lesions on the skin surface. The swellings may persist for a few hours or a few days. Among common causes are allergies to drugs, insect stings or bites, or certain foods. Eggs, fruits, nuts, and shellfish are often causes of skin reactions in sensitive persons. Some foods can produce reactions after only small amounts are consumed. Others, particularly strawberries, seem to result in urticaria only after an excessive amount has been eaten. Histamine often is involved in the reaction and antihistamines frequently reduce the symptoms.

USP unit A standard of potency of a substance as established by the United States Pharmacopeial Convention, composed of physicians and scientists, and published in the *United States Pharmacopeia* (U.S.P.). The U.S.P. is the legally recognized reference work on the strength, purity, and other quality factors of drugs and related substances in the United States by terms of the U.S. Food, Drugs, and Cosmetic Act. Other countries publish similar official reference works for standards of medicines and related materials and identified by abbreviations, such as B.P. for *British Pharmacopeia.*

U.S. RDA The Recommended Daily Allowances established by the U.S. Food and Drug Administration for the nutrient requirements listed on labels of foods and vitamin preparations. For most nutrients they are the highest figures recommended in the recommended dietary allowances tables for all males and females above the age of 3 years, with exceptions made for pregnant or nursing mothers who require additional amounts of some nutrients. See *recommended dietary allowances.*

V

vaccination The introduction of a vaccine into the body in order to produce immunity to a particular disease. The vaccine is composed of the bodies of microorganisms, such as bacteria, rickettsiales, or viruses, that cause the disease. The body's immune system reacts to the vaccine in the same way it would respond to an invasion by the disease organism itself by developing antibodies to resist a future attack by the organism. The term is derived from the Latin word for cow, *vacca*, because the first vaccine was developed from cowpox for the purpose of protecting people from smallpox, a related disease.

valine One of the essential amino acids. It is required for normal growth in children and for nitrogen balance in adults. An infant requires more than 6 times as much valine as an adult but the daily requirement declines sharply during the first 10 years of life. Sources include wheat gluten, whole eggs, peanut flour, brewer's yeast, casein, fish, wheat germ, egg albumin, and soybean meal, in addition to meat, poultry, fish, and dairy products.

vanadium A mineral essential in small quantities for the normal life functions of most animals. Daily requirements for humans are uncertain but laboratory animals deprived of vanadium show signs of retarded growth, particularly impaired bone development, and defects in reproductive function and fat metabolism.

vegans A term for individuals who eat only foods from plant sources; all animal foods in any form are avoided. Sometimes called *pure vegetarians*, it is this group whose members may develop a vitamin B-12 deficiency unless the vitamin is obtained from a source like yeast or a B-12 supplement. See *vegetarians; vitamin B-12*.

vegetarians Those people whose food source is primarily of plant origin. They are divided into three groups: *ovo-lactovegetarians*, or those who do not eat meat, but use milk, milk products, and eggs; *lactovegetarians*, or those who refrain from eating meat and eggs; and *vegans*, pure vegetarians. See *vegans*.

Violet No. 1 One of several FD&C synthetic colors that has been "delisted" or banned from the U.S. Food and Drug Administration's list of authorized food additives. It was banned in 1973 because a study showed an association between the dye and cancer in rats, although the dye had been used for 22 years without evidence of ill effects in humans. The rats that developed cancer were fed a diet in which 5 percent of the meal was Violet No. 1.

viosterol Ergocalciferol in solution in a neutral oil. See entries under *ergocalciferol; vitamin D*.

viruses Very tiny disease agents that are much smaller than bacteria and sometimes consist of little more than a DNA molecule. A virus does not require a metabolic system or the usual substances of a tissue cell because it is a parasite that uses the materials of the cell it invades. A typical virus takes control of the cell it invades and forces the cell's metabolic machinery to manufacture additional viruses; the cell soon bursts and releases a new generation of viruses to invade other body cells. Most viruses are not affected by antibiotics, so viral infections are difficult to control. They are responsible for numerous diseases, including mumps, mononucleosis, herpes, and measles.

visual purple A protein-based pigment in the retina of the eye that is sensitive to light. When light falls on the pigment, it is bleached to another pigment, sometimes called *visual yellow*. The energy transfer from the light to the pigment results in the visual image that is transmitted to the brain by way of the optic nerve, which extends its fibers into the retina. Vitamin A is a component of visual purple, which is rebuilt during periods when the eye is not exposed to light; however, new daily supplies of vitamin A are required to maintain the visual purple function. A lack of vitamin A results in night blindness and other disorders of vision in poor light conditions. Also called *rhodopsin*.

visual violet See *iodopsin*.

vitamin Any of a group of organic chemical compounds generally present in foods and necessary for one or more vital body functions. A deficiency of a vitamin results in symptoms or signs of a disease condition.

Substances identified as vitamins usually cannot be synthesized by the human body, although in some cases the same chemical can be synthesized by other organisms, including "friendly bacteria" that live in the human digestive tract. Some vitamins may be produced by body tissues but at rates that are not great enough to meet the body's own needs and must be supplemented by foods or vitamin supplements. Most foods contain more than one vitamin, but no single food is an adequate source of all the vitamins required by people. Many vitamins do not enter directly into the composition of body tissues but merely serve as catalysts to aid the body in carrying out certain physiological activities. However, they are eventually consumed, converted, or excreted and must be replaced on a more or less daily basis. This is particularly true of the water-soluble vitamins that are regularly washed out of the body in waste fluids. Fat-soluble vitamins remain in the body tissues for longer periods, but sooner or later must be replaced like any other nutrient.

Vitamins were discovered somewhat accidentally by scientists in a series of experiments beginning around 1880. It was found that when laboratory animals were provided with diets of pure proteins, fats, carbohydrates, and essential minerals, or fed meals that contained all the known components of milk, they became sick and died. However, animals on the purified diets recovered when they were also given a few drops of fresh milk each day. Obviously, the researchers concluded, there is something in food besides mere chemical compounds that is needed to sustain life. But some 30 years elapsed before other scientists found that milk, butter, and egg yolk contained traces of substances, some soluble in water and some soluble in fats or fat solvents, that were necessary for normal growth and longevity. At first the unidentified substances were called *food hormones*. Then, in 1912, a Polish expatriate, Casimir Funk, studying the causes of Oriental beriberi, found a similar food hormone in the bran removed from rice. Funk suggested, since the substance appeared to be related to amino acids, that all food hormones be called *vitamines*, meaning the "amines of life." Later, it was found that not all such substances were amines and it was agreed to drop the "e" from *vitamine*, but the somewhat inappropriate name has been accepted by everyone since then. Although vitamins were originally designated by letters of the alphabet, recent research has found that some vitamins occur in more than one form, some are more easily recognized by a chemical or other name, and some substances once identified as vitamins were found not to be vitamins at all. Thus, all vitamins today have at least two names, one identifying the substance by a letter of the alphabet and one identifying it by a chemical name. See the specific entry.

vitamin A   A fat-soluble vitamin, *retinol*, that occurs in two different forms in nature and can also be manufactured by the human body from provitamins in the diet.

Despite their differences, the two basic forms of vitamin A—sometimes identified as vitamin A-1 and vitamin A-2—have virtually the same effects on the human body. Vitamin A-1 is the type people acquire by eating milk, butter, liver, or egg yolk. Vitamin A-2 is present in fresh-water fish and in birds that eat fresh-water fish. The provitamins are the *carotenes*, the yellow to reddish-orange plant pigments of such fruits and vegetables as apricots, carrots, corn, and peaches. The carotenes provide vitamin A to humans through a process of molecule splitting that occurs in the liver and in the wall of the small intestine. One of the carotenes, for example, is converted into two molecules of vitamin A for each carotene molecule.

Vitamin A is so named because it was the first of the fat-soluble vitamins to be discovered and was known originally as *fat-soluble A factor*. When other fat-soluble vitamins were found by scientists, fat-soluble A became simply *vitamin A*. The A-vitamin was discovered almost by accident during experiments in the early twentieth century at the University of Wisconsin where researchers were using rats to test different combinations of grains and fodders that could be used for feeding cattle. It had been observed that animals provided with green fodder seemed to thrive better than those given only grain. More interesting, however, was an experiment in which a small change was made in the diet of rats that had been fed a presumably perfect diet of balanced nutrients, using butter as the source of fats. The ideal diet was continued except that lard was substituted for butter. Within 3 months the once-normal, healthy rats had become blind and were dying. When butter was returned to their diet, the rats' health was restored. Other fats were tested. Fish oil had the restorative effect of butter but olive oil caused the type of blindness that occurred when lard was the source of fat. Thus, around 1910, scientists became aware that a substance present in certain fats, but not all fats, was essential to normal health. Another 10 years passed before other researchers found the link between carotene and vitamin A, although they had been aware that certain green leaves produced a benefit similar to that of the substance in butter and fish oil.

As often happens, empirical evidence—the knowledge acquired by personal experience as distinguished from scientific knowledge—precedes the evidence acquired by logic and experiment. Witches treated heart disease with foxglove before doctors discovered digitalis, the active ingredient of foxglove, and Hindus used snakeroot as a tranquilizer for 2,500 years before western doctors found that snakeroot contained reserpine, an antihypertension drug. So also did Europeans in the Middle Ages know that eating liver would prevent night blindness. But not until the twentieth century did medical researchers discover that vitamin A, which is found in liver, would prevent night blindness. The reason vitamin A prevents night blindness is related to the other effects of the vitamin on vision. The eye is probably more sensitive to a vitamin A deficiency than other organs because the vitamin enters into the function of sight. Vitamin A, in either of its forms, is united in the retina of the eye with a protein in a substance called *rhodopsin*, or *visual purple*.

Visual purple is a light-sensitive pigment. It absorbs the energy of light entering the eye and striking the retina, translating the energy patterns formed by the image on the retina into nerve impulses that are carried back from the retina and along the optic nerve to the visual centers of the brain. Visual purple loses its potency after a period of time and becomes bleached. The bleached version of the substance is called *visual yellow*. At night, when the eye is usually resting, visual yellow is restored to visual purple by returning the vitamin A portion to the molecule. For this to take place, a certain amount of fresh vitamin A is required each day. Before vitamin A is depleted, when the amount consumed each day is less than the amount used, the deficiency begins to make itself felt in a condition called *dark adaptation,* in which a person has difficulty adjusting to the diminished light in a darkened room. The effect also shows up as night blindness, a variation of dark adaptation caused by a very low level of visual purple. The individual's retinal cells have enough of the visual pigment to see things in good light but not enough for vision in poor light. If the condition is recognized early enough, normal vision in dim light can usually be restored by ingestion of vitamin A. If vitamin A intake is not increased, however, the person becomes progressively blind.

Vitamin A is also essential for the growth and maintenance of tissues of the skin and the membranes lining the digestive, genitourinary, and respiratory organs. A vitamin A deficiency is particularly critical for young persons who may experience a variety of ill effects ranging from stunted growth to a failure of the teeth to develop a normal layer of enamel. A deficiency at any stage of life can result in a dry, scaly skin, an eye inflammation called *xerophthalmia,* and a deterioration of the mucous membranes characterized by increased susceptibility to sore throat, sinus infections, salivary gland infections, and systemic infections that can enter the bloodstream through damaged linings of the digestive tract.

Fortunately, because vitamin A is fat soluble it can be stored in the body, mostly in the liver. It is released into the bloodstream at a fairly constant rate, so the effects of a vitamin A deficiency develop rather slowly. The amount of vitamin A reserves in the body tissues of any individual vary with a number of factors, including the person's intake of vitamin A or provitamin A foods during previous weeks and months. Certain health conditions can also influence one's vitamin A stores; cirrhosis of the liver hampers the ability of that organ to supply vitamin A. The vitamin A content of butterfat is higher during the summer when cows feed on fresh green vegetation than in winter. Vegetarians require a larger intake of carotene sources than people who eat butter, milk, and liver. However, some animals store so much vitamin A in their livers that eating large amounts of liver over long periods can result in vitamin A toxicity, or *hypervitaminosis.* Headache, nausea, diarrhea, and loss of bone calcium are symptoms of hypervitaminosis A. However, there seems to be no evidence of serious illness from consuming an excess of carotene; unabsorbed carotene is excreted in the feces. The only strange effect of excess carotene seems to be an accumulation of yellow pigment in the skin.

vitamin activity A measure of the value of a specific food in terms of its content of a vitamin or vitamins.

vitamin antagonist Any substance that interferes with the normal action of a vitamin in body functions. One example is the antituberculosis drug, isoniazid, which interferes with the function of vitamin B-6, or pyridoxine, in human tissues. Raw fish contains an enzyme, thiaminase, that destroys vitamin B-1, or thiamine. Also called *antivitamin.*

vitamin B   See *B-complex vitamins.*

vitamin B-1   See *thiamine.*

vitamin B-2   See *riboflavin.*

vitamin B-5   See *niacin.*

vitamin B-6   See *pyridoxal; pyridoxamine; pyridoxine.*

vitamin B-12   A vitamin of the B-complex that is unique in that it contains a metallic element, cobalt, which is the reason for the vitamin's alternative name, *cobalamin.* Vitamin B-12 is important because of its role in the normal production of red blood cells and the maintenance of a healthy nervous system. It has been associated for a number of years with a condition known as *pernicious anemia* and a number of disorders, such as the *malabsorption syndromes.*

The relationship between the liver, a source of vitamin B-12, and pernicious anemia was discovered in 1926. But more than 20 years elapsed before the vitamin was isolated from the liver, which helps explain the effectiveness of liver extract as a treatment for pernicious anemia. As in other vitamin history puzzles, livestock growers had been aware for years that cattle and sheep that grazed in pastures where the soil lacked cobalt did not thrive and, in fact, frequently became victims of disease. But the best medical minds of the day could not believe that a lack of cobalt in the soil could account for diseases in livestock. Even harder to believe at first was a later discovery that a strain of *Streptomyces* bacteria in the digestive tract could manufacture a vitamin that could prevent pernicious anemia. The adult human requires only miniscule amounts of vitamin B-12, about 1 μg or a bit more is usually sufficient. A microgram is approximately 1/30,000,000 of 1 oz. A pernicious anemia patient around the year 1930 was required to eat as much as 8 oz. of liver a day to get that amount of vitamin B-12 into his system and would appreciate the fact that a modern vitamin tablet provides that amount and much more in the way of nutrients.

However, pernicious anemia is a little more complicated than a simple problem of vitamin B-12 deficiency. It depends on an *intrinsic factor* and an *extrinsic factor*; with the vitamin acting as extrinsic factor because it involves a substance produced outside the body tissues. The intrinsic factor is produced inside the body tissues, in the lining of the stomach in a normal person. It binds itself to the extrinsic factor, vitamin B-12, and escorts it through the wall of the small intestine. If the stomach lining cells do not secrete the intrinsic factor, vitamin B-12 is not absorbed. People whose stomachs do not produce the intrinsic factor, which is a heat-sensitive protein molecule, are susceptible to pernicious anemia. The condition is believed to be inherited.

The vitamin B-12 molecule is very similar to the heme portion of the hemoglobin molecule of red blood cells and apparently this relationship contributes to this vitamin's role in helping the body produce normal red blood cells. In addition to this role, vitamin B-12 performs other functions, such as the formation of DNA and RNA molecules and working with pantothenic acid to rearrange atoms within amino acids when new ones are manufactured from parts of others. A lack of vitamin B-12 due to absence of the intrinsic factor can result in a progressive degeneration of tracts of the spinal cord, a condition known as *posterolateral sclerosis*. The patient loses the sense of touch and pain and experiences a loss of his sense of position in space, with gradual muscular wasting and increasing mental changes, leading to death within 2 years. However, the disorder responds almost miraculously to vitamin B-12 treatments, which can restore the person to good health indefinitely—although any nerve damage caused before vitamin B-12 treatments is usually permanent and cannot be reversed.

Vitamin B-12 is found almost exclusively in animal food sources and some are better than others. Beef liver is the richest source of B-12 and contains an average of twice as much of the vitamin as the next best source, beef kidney, and nearly 10 times as much as a beef steak. Muscle meats, fish, and milk are moderately good sources, but a serving of ham or fish will provide only the minimum intake of about 1 μg. A typical serving of cereal grains or vegetables will provide about 1/10 of 1 μg. of vitamin B-12. People who are strict vegans risk development of the nervous system symptoms of vitamin B-12 deficiency, but may be protected against anemia if they consume adequate amounts of folic acid from grains and vegetables. Vitamin B-12 deficiencies can be caused by a variety of disorders other than lack of the intrinsic factor. Malabsorption syndromes, such as sprue, tapeworms, pancreatic insufficiency, and digestive tract abnormalities like diverticula and blind loops can interfere with absorption of vitamin B-12. Even among normal people, the percentage of vitamin B-12 absorbed can be as little as one-half the amount contained in the diet because of various metabolic and physiological factors, so a person may need to plan an intake of about 2 μg. per day in order to be fairly certain of getting 1 μg. of vitamin B-12 into the bloodstream.

vitamin B-15   See *pangamic acid*.

vitamin B-17   See *amygdalin*.

vitamin B-C   See *folic acid*.

vitamin B-t   See *carnitine*.

vitamin B-x   See *para-aminobenzoic acid*.

vitamin C   The common name for *ascorbic acid*, the antiscurvy vitamin found in many fruits and vegetables, particularly citrus fruits, and also manufactured synthetically. The vitamin designation replaced an earlier term of *water-soluble C*, the third in the series of nutrient factors after *fat-soluble A* and *water-soluble B* in the history of vitamin discoveries. Vitamin C is the only water-soluble vitamin that does not contain nitrogen in its molecule. The molecular structure itself is a very simple sugar-like unit of carbon, hydrogen, and oxygen atoms. It is also very unstable, being sensitive to the effects of air, heat, alkalis, and may even react with certain metals, such as the copper in cooking utensils.

The need to maintain an adequate level of vitamin C in the body by eating certain foods is a problem peculiar to only a few species of animals, including humans, monkeys, guinea pigs, and an Oriental bat that eats fruit. Other animals synthesize ascorbic acid in their bodies. The vitamin is best known today for its effects in preventing scurvy, which is one of the oldest nutritional diseases known to man. Hippocrates, the ancient Greek physician, described scurvy nearly 2,500 years ago. The disease was a sort of calculated risk for people who traveled far from home, as noted in the records of the crusades during the eleventh to thirteenth centuries and of the early sea explorations; during one brief period of the sixteenth century, England lost 10,000 sailors to scurvy. Because vitamin C contributes to a kind of cement that holds body cells together, an ascorbic acid deficiency is usually marked by bleeding, spongy gums and loose teeth, and tender and swollen joints. Bleeding is common beneath the skin and the mucous membranes and around the bones and joints. Sometimes the leg pains are misdiagnosed as rheumatism. Small children are particularly vulnerable because heated milk formulas and infant cereals lack vitamin C or provide inadequate amounts. Small children deprived of vitamin C often show retarded growth, irritability, and restlessness, in addition to the usual scurvy symptoms. Cases of subacute scurvy have been found in homes where infants were provided with orange-flavored soda which the mothers believed, incorrectly, to be the same as pure orange juice.

Besides preventing scurvy, vitamin C is involved in the metabolism of at least two amino acids and in the function of folic acid, a member of the vitamin B-complex. It also increases the availability to the body of iron contained in the diet by making it easier for the iron to be absorbed from the digestive tract. It is vital to the formation of fibrous and connective tissues of the body, in the structure of blood capillaries, and in the formation of teeth and bones. Vitamin C is essential for the normal functioning of an enzyme that is involved in building new cell walls, and it appears to enable the body to withstand injury from burns and bacterial poisons.

Although scurvy has been recognized for thousands of years and people have probably known for just as long of remedies to treat the symptoms, the exact role of vitamin C was not discovered until the 1930s. Ironically, ascorbic acid had been extracted from citrus fruits several years earlier but scientists did not recognize the substance immediately as the *antiscorbutic*, or *antiscurvy*, factor because it had not been tested for that purpose. British admirals were aware of the need to carry oranges and lemons on long sea voyages nearly 150 years before the physician James Lind made the same recommendation, for which he is honored as the person who discovered the need for citrus fruits to prevent scurvy. Also, unwittingly, both sailors and landlubbers seemed aware that drinking beer helped to prevent the disease. It was not the type of beer served today in bottles or metal containers, but a sort of homemade brew prepared from freshly sprouted barley. The sprouts, it is now known, can be a source of vitamin C. Legume sprouts, as used in Oriental dishes, also contain vitamin C, although it is not available in the dried or cooked forms of these vegetables. Ship captains of past centuries often requested that among the men aboard there should be at least one person with a knowledge of making home brew. It might be noted that when the *Mayflower* approached the New England coast in 1620, the ship stopped at what is now Provincetown, on Cape Cod, to make a fresh batch of beer before sailing on to Plymouth Rock. A folk remedy for scurvy also used in the past was a tea made of pine needles. American Indians and natives of northern Europe were familiar with the benefits of pine needle tea when citrus fruits, barley beer, or other sources of vitamin C were not available. Pine needle tea also prevented outbreaks of scurvy among wagon-train pioneers heading west in the nineteenth century.

Except for vitamin C tablets, orange juice is probably the most convenient way of getting one's daily requirements of ascorbic acid. The minimum daily requirement is 30 mg. of vitamin C. The recommended dietary allowance is 70 mg. per day, with dose levels of up to 100 mg. per day sometimes advised for adolescent children, pregnant women, and nursing mothers. A 6-oz. glass of fresh orange juice provides 93 mg. of vitamin C, which is approximately the maximum recommended daily dose. Other natural sources—all fresh fruits and fresh vegetables or minimally cooked vegetables—include strawberries, grapefruit or grapefruit juice, lemons or lemon juice, cantaloupe, honeydew melon, watermelon, and most berries; kale leaves, turnip greens, green peppers, broccoli, Brussels sprouts, mustard greens, collards, cauliflower, spinach, cabbage, rutabagas, asparagus, and tomatoes or tomato juice. All of these foods provide on the average of 20 mg. or more of vitamin C per serving. Fruits with the lowest levels of vitamin C per average serving include apples, pears, grapes, and plums. Onions, radishes, and cooked string beans are the poorest vegetable sources of vitamin C.

Certain pigments and other parts of citrus fruits called *bioflavonoids* are often associated with vitamin C under the heading of vitamin C-complex. Some scientists believe the bioflavonoids hesperidin and rutin play a related role in certain vitamin C functions, such as maintaining integrity of capillary walls. They may serve as vitamin C substitutes or support vitamin C actions in the body. Other bioflavonoids are being studied as well. Although some nutritionists argue that one should eat raw oranges in order to benefit from the bioflavonoids as well as the ascorbic acid, bioflavonoids are available as vitamin supplements for those who for various reasons, such as an allergy to citrus components, may be unable to tolerate raw oranges.

vitamin content The amount of a vitamin in a measured quantity of food, such as a 100-g. or 3.5-oz. serving. The amount is usually indicated in micrograms (1 µg. equals about 1/30,000,000 of 1 oz.) or in international units (IU).

vitamin D A fat-soluble vitamin that occurs in several forms in nature and can be manufactured in the body from provitamins. The primary function of vitamin D is to regulate the absorption and utilization of calcium in the diet for the purpose of building and maintaining the bones and teeth. Vitamin D also enhances the absorption of phosphorus from the intestine and its use by the body in skeletal tissues. A deficiency of vitamin D results in bone abnormalities, particularly the childhood disease known as *rickets*. Similar bone defects with other names can occur later in life because of vitamin D-related calcium deficiencies.

Vitamin D is sometimes called the "sunshine vitamin" because ultraviolet light of the sun, and also artificial ultraviolet light sources, convert provitamin substances in the skin of people and animals into vitamin D. A deficiency of vitamin D is most likely to occur in the absence of sunlight, as during the winter months in areas remote from the equator, and in persons whose skin is protected from exposure to sunlight by clothing in milder climates.

There are about a dozen substances that can be converted into vitamin D by ultraviolet light, but only two are important in human health. One that occurs mainly in plants is called *ergosterol* and is converted to vitamin D-2. The other is a type of cholesterol and is converted by sunlight into vitamin D-3. The D-3 form of the vitamin is the type associated with fish oils, such as cod-liver oil. However, a dietary source of vitamin D is usually necessary to prevent a deficiency of the vitamin because a majority of people beyond the tropics are usually unable to absorb enough sunlight throughout the year to convert the provitamins that may be in the skin. In northern cities, for example, dust and smoke pollution of the atmosphere can block the ultraviolet rays of the sun from reaching the surface of the earth, even when the weather is mild enough to permit exposure of a large area of skin surface for a long period. When sunbathing is possible in almost any climate, people who are light skinned usually apply a suntan lotion to their skin; the purpose of the sunscreen or lotion is to block the ultraviolet rays of the sun. The alternative, of course, is to risk a severe sunburn. People whose skins are naturally dark are protected from the sun's rays by their skin pigment, which also prevents the ultraviolet light from activating provitamin D. In fact, studies show that a dark-skinned person living in a northern industrial city is at the greatest risk of suffering a vitamin D deficiency—unless his daily diet contains an adequate amount of vitamin D. Once vitamin D is absorbed by the small intestine, it is diffused through the body's lymphatic system and the body's tissues cannot tell the difference between vitamin D manufactured in the skin from vitamin D in cod-liver oil, a vitamin D additive in breakfast cereal, or the vitamin D in a vitamin tablet.

Vitamin D deficiency as manifested by rickets is another of the many diseases that has plagued humans for centuries. The very name rickets is inherited from the Greek word *rhachitis*, meaning a bone disorder. During the seventeenth century, some doctors called rickets the "English sickness" because it was prevalent among children of the English industrial cities where coal smoke blotted out what little sunlight was available. But not all children of England and neighboring areas suffered from the disease. Those who lived along the coastal regions could dine on herring, cod, mackerel, or other fish that contained oils rich in vitamin D. At times people living in inland areas of northern Europe suspected that something in oily fish protected against bone deformities and tried to obtain the fish for their children. Scientific knowledge at that time did not include even a dream that invisible substances in fish oil might protect against rickets, and doctors for many years discouraged parents from giving salt-water fish oils to their children. Like other effective remedies that they did not understand, physicians branded the fish oil as just another example of witchcraft and superstition.

Interest by doctors in fish oils as a source of an antirickets substance was revived during World War I when a series of coincidences in Europe made vitamin D the answer to a centuries-old puzzle. The war had increased the incidence of rickets through food shortages and doctors who believed rickets was caused by a contagious disease began sending children to sunny climates to recover. At about the same time, the ultraviolet lamp was invented and doctors noted that it had the same effect on rickets as a trip to the Mediterranean area. Meanwhile, a British scientist trying to find a cure for dogs crippled by rickets added fish oil to their usual diet of oatmeal and milk. The dogs not only recovered but resumed their normal growth rate. Still another researcher had just discovered that rats deprived of either calcium or phosphorus seemed to recover from symptoms of rickets when given fish oil. Suddenly all the pieces of the puzzle fell into place: The fish oil, ultraviolet light, and calcium and phosphorus intake were all a part of the same picture of rickets. The substance in the fish oil was named vitamin D in 1922. Within a few years, the provitamins converted to vitamin D by ultraviolet light had been identified, and by the end of that decade, nutrition experts had also developed a method of irradiating milk, bread, and other foods with ultraviolet light. Vitamin D-enriched foods are generally available today in all areas and seasons.

Other food sources of vitamin D include beef and pork liver, liver sausage, beefsteak, egg yolks, shrimp and most salt-water fish, butter, cheese, and cream. Except for carrot tops, corn oil, and a few other vegetable items, vegetarian sources are usually not significant as sources of vitamin D.

A deficiency of vitamin D results in a failure of the intestine to absorb adequate amounts of calcium and phosphorus from food items. Those minerals are excreted in the urine in the absence of vitamin D and blood levels fall, particularly levels of phosphorus. The body's chemistry mechanisms then begin to "shave" calcium and phosphorus from the bones. In adults, the condition is called *osteomalacia*, or softening of the bone. In children, the effect is rickets and is more serious because the bones are still developing. Children with rickets experience bowleg, knock-knee, spinal curvature, and teeth that are poorly formed and susceptible to decay. An excess of vitamin D results in a toxic condition marked by loss of appetite, vomiting, diarrhea, headache, drowsiness, and increased thirst and urine production.

Vitamin D deficiencies can occur in spite of adequate levels of vitamin D and calcium and phosphorus intake because of digestive tract disorders, such as celiac-sprue, which interfere with the absorption of fats. The use of mineral oil medications can also interfere with vitamin D effectiveness by blocking the absorption of the vitamin and organic fats in the digestive tract.

vitamin derivative   A chemical compound produced in the body from vitamins, vitamin components, or provitamins.

vitamin E   A fat-soluble vitamin that occurs in four different forms, all identified as a tocopherol with a Greek-letter prefix. The various forms—alpha-, beta-, gamma-, and delta-tocopherol—differ mainly in the positions and numbers of atoms in their molecular structures. All are viscous oils that are stable with heat but sensitive to ultraviolet light (including sunlight) and oxygen. Their main function appears to be an antioxidant role, preventing the oxidation of unsaturated fatty acids in the body tissues as fats become rancid when oxidized. The alpha-form of vitamin E is the most active of the four tocopherols.

Vitamin E is associated with a reproductive function because of early experiments with laboratory rats which showed that a deficiency of the substance resulted in degeneration of the male sex tissues and immobilization of the spermatozoa. In the female, a vitamin E deficiency caused spontaneous abortion and fetal death of offspring. In other animals, a lack of vitamin E was found to be associated with fluid retention, progressive muscular dystrophy, excretion of creatine (a substance important as an energy storehouse), and softening of the brain. In humans, certain digestive disorders, particularly those associated with the gall bladder and pancreas, have been found to respond to vitamin E treatments. It has also been used effectively in treating certain blood and skin disorders of newborn infants. It is believed that vitamin E also protects the vitamin A stores in fatty tissues and is necessary for the prevention of oxidation of unsaturated fatty acids that are components of red blood cells and brain tissues.

Wheat germ is one of the richest sources of tocopherols, a fact that was unknown in the 1920s when scientists found that a deficiency of vitamin E could cause sterility in rats. At that time, consumers demanded white bread. Dark breads were shunned by customers in many Western industrialized nations. Some bakeries stopped offering whole-wheat bread because there was no demand. The flour manufacturers were pleased because pure white flour could be produced without the risk of a rancid flavor that can develop in flour containing wheat germ. When nutrition experts of the era determined that something was lacking in the food value of white bread, it was decided that thiamine, or vitamin B-1, could be added. The knowledge that whole-wheat flour contains more thiamine than "vitamin-enriched" white flour was ignored. Today, whole-wheat flour and wheat germ have regained their acceptability, partly because of the publicity surrounding the rat sterility studies, which suggested a risk of loss of sexual potency from eating pure white flour, and more recent findings of possible nerve and muscle disorders associated with a vitamin E deficiency.

Other sources of vitamin E are corn, cottonseed, and soybean oils, margarines, eggs, fish, liver and other meats, and butter. Fruits and vegetables generally are not good sources, and commercial processing and storage of some foods reduces vitamin E content. Vitamin E is usually resistant to cooking but can be destroyed by deep-fat frying. Absorption of vitamin E from foods can be hindered by use of mineral-oil remedies and digestive disorders, such as cystic fibrosis, biliary tract diseases, and malabsorption syndromes, including celiac disease.

vitamin F   See *essential fatty acid*.

vitamin G   See *riboflavin*.

vitamin H   See *biotin*.

vitamin K   A generic term for a group of fat-soluble vitamins that enhances blood-clotting activity by increasing the synthesis of prothrombin, one of the dozen factors involved in the body's complicated process of blood coagulation.

The vitamin acquired the letter "K" designation because it was first discovered in Denmark in 1935 and identified as the *Koagulation* factor. Scientists in North America and other parts of the world simply followed the Danish spelling and adopted the first letter of the word as the vitamin's common name. Like some other vitamins, vitamin K was discovered during animal feeding experiments in which the animals died mysteriously while eating a diet that included all known nutrients. The cause of death was a bleeding disease. The animals were newly hatched chicks. And the missing factor, unknown at the time, was a factor present in such diverse foods as hog liver and alfalfa.

The *antihemorrhagic factor* was found to be two different yet quite similar substances. One, now known as *vitamin K-1*, is found in green plant material, such as alfalfa. The second, *vitamin K-2*, is present in certain animal products, such as fish meal. A third, *vitamin K-3*, is a synthetic chemical that is actually more potent than the natural forms of the vitamin and is often used in vitamin supplements under the chemical name of *menadione*, or a *menadiol* compound. Menadione is also the standard used in measuring the potency of vitamin K from natural sources. A number of other substances are also known to have various levels of vitamin K-type activity. The synthetic forms of vitamin K are converted to vitamin K-2 in the body.

The primary function of the K vitamins is in the formation of prothrombin in the liver, the second of 12 stages of blood clotting. Vitamin K is also involved in the synthesis of three other stages of blood clotting. But it serves only as a catalyst and does not actually become incorporated into any of the clot-forming substances. A deficiency of vitamin K results in a reduced level of prothrombin and the ability of the other factors to carry on the various stages of coagulation, leading to a general vulnerability of the individual to losing large quantities of blood from injuries which ordinarily would not be serious. Conditions that interfere with the absorption of fats from the intestine, such as celiac-sprue disease or gall bladder or pancreatic disorders, can also block the absorption of vitamin K and lead to an increased tendency to bleed. Long-term use of internal medications containing mineral oil can interfere with the absorption of any of the fat-soluble vitamins.

Unlike other fat-soluble vitamins, vitamin K is not stored in the body in large quantities. However, the normal intestinal tract contains a friendly strain of bacteria that manufactures vitamin K-2. Vitamin K source foods are mainly green leafy vegetables. The only significant animal source of vitamin K is pork liver; milk and eggs contain small amounts. The richest sources of the vitamin are spinach, cauliflower, and cabbage, each of which contains more vitamin K per 3-oz. serving than pork liver, and from 50 to 60 times as much per equal-size serving as milk. Other relatively good sources are carrots, potatoes, soybeans, wheat germ, wheat bran, green and ripe tomatoes, and strawberries.

Newborn infants are particularly vulnerable to vitamin K deficiencies because they have not yet had time to develop the normal human culture of intestinal bacteria that produces the vitamin. For that reason, newborn infants and mothers in labor are often administered therapeutic doses of vitamin K. Therapeutic doses of vitamin K may also be recommended for persons who take anticoagulant drugs, such as dicoumarol, which is a vitamin K antagonist. For most healthy persons, very small amounts of vitamin K are needed, amounts that are measured in micrograms, levels so small that it takes more than 30 million to make 1 oz.

The trace mineral manganese is associated with vitamin K, serving as a cofactor in prothrombin formation. A deficiency of manganese sometimes accompanies a deficiency of vitamin K in humans.

vitamin M   See *folic acid.*

vitamin P   See *bioflavonoids*.

vitamin potency   The amount of a vitamin in a vitamin supplement, usually expressed in RDAs or MDRs.

vitamin precursors   Compounds that can be converted within an organism into the active form of the vitamin, such as beta-carotene to vitamin A, or tryptophan to niacin. Also called *provitamins*.

vitamin-related compounds   Substances that are similar in some reactions to vitamins, but their need in human nutrition has not been established. See *coenzyme*.

vitamin supplements   Vitamins that are available in tablet, capsule, or liquid form, with or without a doctor's prescription. A supplement may contain a variety of vitamins plus certain essential minerals and may be recommended for persons suffering from or recovering from an illness or injury, people on severe weight-control or physician-prescribed diets whose food intake may limit availability of vitamins from natural sources, elderly individuals, pregnant women or nursing mothers, and children.

vitamin T   See *torutilin*.

vitamin toxicity   The adverse health effects of consuming excessive doses of vitamins on a regular basis. This condition is most likely to occur with overdoses of fat-soluble vitamins, which tend to be retained by the tissues longer than water-soluble vitamins. Vitamin A toxicity is characterized by skin disorders and loss of hair, headaches, visual defects, loss of appetite, and a tendency to bleed easily. Vitamin D toxicity is marked by accumulation of calcium in the tissues, particularly the kidneys, which may be damaged permanently.

vitamin U   See *metenoic acid*.

W

walking exercise A form of physical activity often recommended as a basic form of exercise in which nearly anybody can participate for the improvement of respiratory, circulatory, muscular and weight benefits. The amount of energy required for walking depends on the weight of the individual and the walking speed, as well as the slope of the terrain. An 80-lb. person walking at 2 mph uses less than 2 calories per minute, whereas a 200-lb. person walking at a speed of 4 mph burns 7 calories per minute. For a 155-lb. person walking up an inclined path, caloric expenditure rises to 9 per minute. The average adult walking at a pace of 2 to 3 mph burns about 4 calories per minute.

water A clear, odorless, tasteless liquid that is essential for normal health. The human body is approximately 60 percent water, with an average daily input-output balance of about 2.5 qt.

Next to oxygen, water is the most important substance in the environment; a human can live only a very few days without a fresh supply of water to replace the amount lost through urine, feces, sweat, and water vapor from the lungs. The need for water is more important for an infant than an adult. An infant body may be as much as 75 percent water with a daily turnover that is nearly 3 times that of an adult's needs when figured on a basis of ounces of water per pound of body weight. A human can lose all the carbohydrates and fats in his body and still survive, but a loss of 20 percent of body water can be fatal. With an adequate supply of fresh water, a human can live for several days without solid food by using his own body tissues as a source of nutrients.

About 1 gal. of water is used by the body as fluid for blood circulation. That water helps carry nutrients to tissue cells throughout the body and removes the waste products of cell metabolism. Minerals and other substances are transported in water in a dissolved state. Substances that become electrolytes when dissolved in water are able to cross cell membranes and participate in metabolic activities. The protoplasm of the cells where metabolism occurs is about 75 percent water. Still another function of water in the body is that of heat regulation. Water not only helps carry excess body heat to the surface where it can be dispersed but a significant amount reaches the outside of the skin where it helps cool the body by evaporation, a process commmonly known as perspiration or sweating.

water balance The normal state of the body in which about 60 percent of the body weight is water which is distributed so that two-thirds is held in the tissue cells and one-third in extracellular fluids, such as blood and lymph. In normal water balance, fluid input equals fluid output and ranges between 2 and 3 qt. per day for the average adult. More than half of fluid intake is in the form of liquids; the remainder comes from water contained in solid foods and water produced by metabolic activity. Urine accounts for about half of fluid output each day; the remainder is in feces, sweat, and water vapor exhaled from the lungs.

water intoxication A disorder of water balance. If an individual for whatever reason has a water intake that exceeds the body's ability to excrete water, a toxic condition can develop. Symptoms range from loss of appetite, weakness, and muscle twitching to delirium and convulsions. Another cause can be the replacement of water after excessive sweating without restoring sodium (salt) loss.

water retention A condition of excess water within the body's cells or in the spaces outside the cells, sometimes marked by water intoxication, circulatory overload, or edema. Water retention may be associated with excessive use of salt, which stimulates the need for water to keep the electrolytes in solution, and with circulatory disorders in which fluid leaks from the blood vessels. See *edema*.

water-soluble vitamins Any vitamins that can be dissolved in water, as distinguished from fat-soluble vitamins, which are not dissolved in water but may be dissolved in fats. Water-soluble vitamins include members of the B-complex and vitamin C. They are easily washed out of the body and are not stored for long periods like fat-soluble vitamins, which can be stored in the body's fat deposits. Because they are water-soluble, the B-complex vitamins are often washed out during cooking and a substantial portion can be lost if the cooking water is discarded.

waxing of foods The practice of coating fruits and vegetables with a thin layer of wax to create an attractive, shiny surface. The wax also helps the produce to retain moisture that otherwise could be lost through evaporation via the pores in the outer surface. The use of wax on fresh produce has been the subject of a health controversy, particularly when applied to the surfaces of items like apples that would be eaten along with the pulp of the fruit.

weight charts The tables of average or ideal weights for people of varying age, height, body build, and sex. Weight charts are compiled by insurance companies, government agencies, and other interested parties for use by individuals in determining how they relate to others of their own types. Because the average weights of adults tend to change from time to time due to such factors as younger generations being larger than older generations at the same age, most weight charts are adjusted periodically. Most health-oriented people use weight charts to monitor their own weight gains or losses in terms of what is considered average or ideal.

weight gain The increase in body weight of an individual. Body weight increases are normal for children or adolescents who are still growing, but weight gains after maturity are a sign of overeating or being physically inactive, or both. The rule-of-thumb for weight gain is that 1 lb. of fat is equivalent to between 3,500 and 3,600 calories. Thus, a person can gain 1 lb. by eating about 3,500 more calories than the body requires, or by curtailing physical activity that would burn approximately 3,500 calories if continued.

weight lifting A form of physical exercise used primarily to develop muscle strength. Weight lifting is not an exercise program in itself because the training does not help develop endurance. Rather, it is considered an adjunct, or addition, to a regular physical exercise program. Weight lifting is usually practiced with barbells or dumbbells, although other equipment can be used as well. Studies show that weight lifting does improve performance in certain other activities, mainly in such sports as the shotput and the broad jump. See *resistance training*.

weight reduction The loss of body weight, or primarily the loss of fat deposits of the body, by exercise, diets, or surgery. For most people, weight reduction can be achieved by a carefully planned decrease in calories accompanied by increased physical activity. Reducing caloric intake is usually more feasible than exercise alone in weight reduction since, for example, one would have to walk 1 mile to burn the calories in one slice of bread. Unsupervised diets require great skill because elimination of foods to reduce calories can also result in the elimination of vital nutrients. Behavior modification through psychotherapy is frequently effective in treating obesity. Surgery is a last resort for massively obese people.

wheat germ The embryo portion of the wheat kernel, which is removed from grain during milling because it is rich in oils that would tend to give the finished flour a rancid taste. The wheat germ, which accounts for only 3 percent of the weight of the wheat kernel, contains the bulk of all the vitamins and other nutrients found in wheat. These include thiamine, niacin, riboflavin, pantothenic acid, vitamins A and E, calcium, phosphorus, iron, and protein; wheat germ is approximately 25 percent protein with a dozen amino acids. Wheat that is milled for use in livestock feed is allowed to retain the wheat germ in the finished product.

whey The fluid by-product of cheese manufacturing. Whey is about 93 percent water and 7 percent lactose and other milk components. Only about half the whey resulting from cheese production is used, mainly in liquid breakfasts, bakery products, ice creams and sherbets, imitation milks, soft drinks, candies, and in the manufacture of vinegar and alcoholic beverages. For each pound of cheese manufactured, about 10 lb. of whey remains; in the United States alone the cheese industry produces about 35 billion lb. of whey each year.

white blood cells Colorless blood corpuscles whose chief purpose is to protect the body against disease. White blood cells have ameboid qualities, meaning they are able to move in directions other than the one followed by the bloodstream. A white blood cell, for example, may take a shortcut directly through the wall of a blood vessel in order to reach an area threatened by injury or infection. There are five main types of white blood cells—basophils, eosinophils, neutrophils, lymphocytes, and monocytes—with specific protective roles. Many white cells attack and consume disease bacteria. Also called *leukocytes*.

whole-grain cereal A cereal in which all parts of the natural cereal kernel are used, as distinguished from regular cereals which are generally made from the starch of the endosperm after the germ and bran have been removed. Regular corn flakes, for example, are made by cooking corn grits (endosperm) to a plastic consistency, rolling the starchy material into flakes, then oven-toasting the flakes.

wound healing The process whereby tissues damaged by accident or surgery heal naturally by gradually closing a gap between several portions with newly formed tissues. A wound usually results in a loss of potassium, sulfur, phosphorus, and amino acids. A clot of fibrin and red blood cells fills the wound at first and serves as a foundation for connective tissue cells that migrate to the fibrin threads and form a matrix for collagen and other tissue materials. The new tissues are invaded by new blood capillaries as healing nears completion. The process requires a diet rich in protein and calories, vitamins C and K, B vitamins, and minerals, particularly calcium.

wrinkles A skin condition caused by tissue changes between the skin's outer layers and the muscle groups below, particularly the loss of fat deposits and the degeneration of elastic connective tissue. Although there are claims that skin wrinkles can be diminished by the use of vitamins or exercises, there is a lack of evidence that such techniques can "cure" wrinkle problems.

X

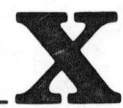

xanthine A purine substance related to nucleic acids that is found in most human body tissues. During processing by the body's chemical mechanisms, xanthine is converted to uric acid which is normally excreted in urine but which can be a cause of gout when it accumulates in the tissues. The xanthines in coffee, tea, and cocoa—caffeine, theophylline, and theobromine—are methylxanthines, a different form of the substance, and are not converted to uric acid.

xanthoma A raised skin lesion, usually yellowish in color, caused by an accumulation of cholesterol under the skin. Xanthomas may range in size from a pinhead to a large nodule and occur most frequently around the eyes, the joints, the neck, or on the palms. The formation of xanthomas is usually a sign of a disorder of fat metabolism and may be associated with diabetes mellitus; a disease of the liver, kidneys, or thyroid gland; or an inherited metabolic disturbance.

xanthurenic acid A substance produced by the metabolism of the amino acid tryptophan. Xanthurenic acid is present in the urine in excessive amounts in people suffering from vitamin B-6 deficiency. The phenomenon is used in a medical test for vitamin B-6 deficiency by giving the patient a dose of tryptophan, measuring 1 g. of the amino acid for each pound of body weight, then measuring the amount of xanthurenic acid in the patient's urine for the next 24 hr.

xerophthalmia A vitamin A deficiency condition characterized by a drying and thickening of the conjunctiva, the thin membrane lining the eyelids, and the surface of the cornea. If the condition is not corrected at an early stage, it may become progressively worse, resulting in blindness. A vitamin A deficiency is also a cause of *night blindness*. See this entry.

xerosis A medical term that refers to an abnormal dryness, as in the vitamin A deficiency disorder of xerophthalmia. The condition can also affect the skin and the mouth.

x-rays The invisible but highly energetic form of electromagnetic radiation used in medical diagnosis and treatment and in food processing. X-rays are used in food processing as an alternative to ultraviolet light to destroy microorganisms, although they are more difficult to focus and control.

Y

yeast The generic name for a group of one-celled fungi that have a rounded shape and reproduce by bud formation. Some kinds of yeast are helpful to humans by aiding in such food processes as baking and brewing whereas others are the cause of infectious diseases, such as moniliasis. Some yeasts are produced as a source of proteins and other nutrients; dry-food yeasts are about one-third protein and are often identified as *single-cell proteins*, or *SCP*. See *baker's yeast; brewer's yeast*.

yeast proteins Proteins obtained from yeast grown on carbohydrates or industrial by-products, such as molasses or cheese whey. After being dried, the yeast may produce as much as one-third extracted protein. The complete yeast cell is more commonly used. See *brewer's yeast*.

yogurt A fermented, custard-like milk product prepared by adding a culture of lactic bacteria to milk—whole, skim, or nonfat—which is the basis of its nutrient value. Also spelled *yoghurt; yoghourt*.

Z

zein A protein of corn lacking in two essential amino acids, tryptophan and lysine, which ranks it as an *incomplete protein*. See this entry; see also *limiting amino acid*.

Zen macrobiotic diet A restrictive dietary method based on a concept that foods can be classified according to an Oriental philosophy of opposing forces called *yin* and *yang*. Brown rice is considered to have the most balanced ratio of these forces. The diet is divided into 10 levels, and though the early levels are well balanced in terms of nutrients, the concept, if carried to an extreme, can lead to life-threatening deficiencies of essential amino acids. Although identified with Zen Buddhism, it is not part of the practice of this religious group.

zinc A mineral needed in small amounts in the human body in order to form a number of enzymes that are involved in important metabolic processes.

Zinc controls the body's levels of vitamin A, the ability of red blood cells to carry away carbon dioxide wastes of breathing, and the metabolism of proteins. Several specific stages of food digestion depend on the availability of zinc in the body. Zinc has been identified as an element associated with the storage of insulin in the pancreas and some studies show this mineral aids in the recovery of body tissues from burns and surgery. A deficiency of zinc is characterized by retarded growth and sexual development due to its role in an enzyme activity important to DNA synthesis and the building of new tissue cells. The senses of taste and smell may be lost as a result of zinc deficiency, and the reduced sensations normally associated with food can in turn cause a loss of appetite and abnormal weight loss. As zinc enhances the recovery from burns and wounds, a deficiency of zinc results in poor recovery from burns and wounds.

A number of factors influence the ability of the human body to absorb zinc from foods in the digestive tract, including the malabsorption syndromes, liver disease, and malnutrition. A substance that binds zinc in the intestine, phytic acid, can reduce absorption; this condition is particularly common in certain

Third World countries where unleavened breads contain a high level of phytic acid compounds. The presence of parasites in the digestive tract can also reduce zinc intake. In Western industrialized countries, kidney dialysis reduces zinc absorption. The best food sources of zinc include oysters, herring, meats, liver, yeast, cereal grains, eggs, and legumes.

zinc:copper ratio The relative proportions of zinc and copper in the diet and body systems. The zinc:copper ratio is believed to play an important role in heart disease because a high-zinc to low-copper proportion is associated with increased cholesterol production by the liver. This theory is also used to explain the fiber relationship in heart disease because fiber binds zinc and reduces its proportion in the ratio. The zinc:copper ratio may further explain the association between hard water and reduced heart disease, as minerals in hard water tend to bind zinc in the digestive tract. Abbreviated *Zn:Cu ratio*.

zymase An enzyme that plays an important role in fermentation processes. It is contained in the yeasts used in alcohol production and related fermentation activities that help preserve foods and make them more digestible by breaking down large, complex nutrient molecules into simpler molecules.

zyme A generic term for something that contributes to fermentation. It was originally a Greek word for *leaven*, meaning to make bread rise. Zyme is generally combined with another word fragment, such as *en* in enzyme, or *lyso*, as in lysozyme, a ferment that breaks down other substances.

Appendix of Tables*

Units of Measure	**227**
Weight, Physical Activity, and Diet	**228**
Recommended Daily Allowances (RDAs) and Nutrient Values of Foods	**232**
Mineral and Vitamin Sources in Foods	**241**

*Source of nutritional data is the U.S. Department of Agriculture.

Units of Measure

Abbreviations*

WEIGHT	LENGTH AND DISTANCE
oz. = ounce	in. = inch
lb. = pound	ft. = foot
g. = gram	cm. = centimeter
kg. = kilogram	m. = meter
mg. = milligram	cm.^{3} = cubic centimeter
µg. = microgram	mph = miles per hour

MEASURE	TEMPERATURE
tsp. = teaspoon	°C = Celsius
tbsp. = tablespoon	°F = Fahrenheit
pt. = pint	
qt. = quart	
fl. oz. = fluid ounce	
ml. = milliliter	

*This table contains an explanation of abbreviated units of measure used in this book.

English–Metric Equivalents

ENGLISH	METRIC
1 ounce (oz.)	28.35 grams (g.)
1 pound (lb.)	454 grams
2.2 pounds	1 kilogram (kg.)
1 inch (in.)	2.54 centimeters (cm.)
39.37 inches	1 meter (m.)
1 cubic inch	16.39 cubic centimeters (cm.^{3})
1 teaspoon (tsp.)	4.9 milliliters (ml.)
1 tablespoon (tbsp.)	14.8 milliliters
1 fluid ounce (fl. oz.)	29.57 milliliters
1 cup	236.6 milliliters
1 pint (pt.)	437.2 milliliters
1 quart (qt.)	946.4 milliliters
1.06 quarts (liquid)	1 liter
0.9 quart (dry)	1 liter

Temperature:

32° Fahrenheit (°F) (freezing)	0° Celsius (°C)
212°Fahrenheit (boiling)	100° Celsius

Gram Equivalents:

1,000 milligrams (mg.)	1 gram (g.)
1,000,000 micrograms (mg.)	1 gram (g.)
1,000 milliliters (ml.)	1 liter (l.)

Weight, Physical Activity, and Diet

Approximate Weights of Adult American Men and Women

HEIGHT WITHOUT SHOES	WEIGHT WITHOUT CLOTHING (POUNDS)		
	Low	*Average*	*High*
Men			
5 ft. 3 in.	118	129	141
5 ft. 4 in.	122	133	145
5 ft. 5 in.	126	137	149
5 ft. 6 in.	130	142	155
5 ft. 7 in.	134	147	161
5 ft. 8 in.	139	151	166
5 ft. 9 in.	143	155	170
5 ft. 10 in.	147	159	174
5 ft. 11 in.	150	163	178
6 ft.	154	167	183
6 ft. 1 in.	158	171	188
6 ft. 2 in.	162	175	192
6 ft. 3 in.	165	178	195
Women			
5 ft.	100	109	118
5 ft. 1 in.	104	112	121
5 ft. 2 in.	107	115	125
5 ft. 3 in.	110	118	128
5 ft. 4 in.	113	122	132
5 ft. 5 in.	116	125	135
5 ft. 6 in.	120	129	139
5 ft. 7 in.	123	132	142
5 ft. 8 in.	126	136	146
5 ft. 9 in.	130	140	151
5 ft. 10 in.	133	144	156
5 ft. 11 in.	137	148	161
6 ft.	141	152	166

How Increasing Physical Activity Helps Balance Caloric Intake

Activities that burn 80 to 100 calories per hour
Reading; writing; eating; watching television; listening to radio; sewing; playing cards; typing; other activities done while sitting that require little or no arm movement.

110 to 160 calories per hour
Preparing and cooking food; washing dishes; dusting; handwashing small articles of clothing; ironing; walking slowly; officework or other activities that are performed while standing.

170 to 240 calories per hour
Mopping; scrubbing; making beds; sweeping; light polishing; waxing; light gardening; carpentry work; walking moderately fast; other activities that are performed while standing and require moderate arm movement; some activities that require vigorous arm movement while sitting.

250 to 350 calories per hour
Vigorous activities, such as heavy scrubbing and waving; handwashing large articles of clothing; hanging out clothes; stripping beds; walking fast; bowling; golfing; heavy gardening work.

350 or more calories per hour
Strenuous activities, such as swimming; playing tennis; bicycling; running or jogging; dancing; skiing; playing other action sports like football or soccer.

Consumption of Sugar Annually per Person in the United States*

FOOD	POUNDS
Cereal and bakery products	17.6
Confectionery products	11.0
Processed fruits and vegetables	10.4
Dairy products	5.8
Other foods (cured meats, etc.)	2.6
Beverages (including soft drinks)	22.8
Total processed foods and beverages	70.2
Household use	24.7
Use in restaurants	5.5
Total per capita sugar consumption	100.2

*By type of use in the 1970s.

Appendix of Tables

Caloric Content of Typical American Snack Foods

FOOD	CALORIES
Candy (except chocolate)	
Caramel; 1 medium	40
Gumdrop; 1 large	40
Jellybeans; 10	105
Peanut brittle; one 2½ X 1½ X 1¼-in. piece; 1 oz.	120
Chocolate	
Bar (sweetened milk chocolate with almonds); 1 oz.	150
Cream; 2 or 3 pieces (35 per pound)	125
Fudge (milk chocolate); 1 piece, 1 to 1½ in. square	115
Chocolate milkshake; 12-oz. glass	515
Mint; 1 piece, 1½ in. in diameter	35
Crackers	
Graham; 2 medium	55
Saltines; 2 crackers, about 2 in. square	25
Doughnut, cake type, 3¼ in. in diameter	165
Popcorn, popped; 1 cup large kernels with added oil and salt	40
Potato chips; 5 medium	60
Pretzels; 5 sticks, about 3 in. long	10

How Adding Fats and Sugar to Foods Changes Their Calorie Count

FOOD	CALORIES
Potatoes	
Boiled, diced, no fat added; ½ cup	55
Mashed, milk and fat added; ½ cup	100
Hash brown; ½ cup	175
French fried; 10 pieces, 3½ to 4 in. long	215
Pan fried; beginning with raw potatoes; ½ cup	230
Peaches; ½ cup	
Fresh, sliced	30
With 2 tsp. sugar	60
With 2 tsp. sugar and ¼ cup half-and-half (milk and cream)	140
Canned	
Water pack	40
Sirup pack	100
Frozen, sweetened	110
Tomato-and-lettuce salad; 1 medium tomato and 2 leaves of lettuce	
Without dressing	25
With 1 tbsp. home-cooked, boiled dressing	50
With 1 tbsp. french dressing	90
With 1 tbsp. commercial salad dressing (mayonnaise type)	90
With 1 tbsp. mayonnaise	125

How Freezing and Canning Foods Changes Their Sodium and Potassium Content*

FOOD	SODIUM	POTASSIUM
Fresh peas	0.9	380.0
Frozen peas	100.0	160.0
Canned peas, without liquid	230.0	180.0

*In milligrams of sodium and potassium per 3.5-oz. serving.

How Nutrient Values of a Potato Can Change with the Form of Preparation

	GRAMS OF POTATO	CALORIES	PROTEIN (GRAMS)	FAT (GRAMS)	CARBOHYDRATE (GRAMS)	IRON (MILLIGRAMS)	VITAMIN C	THIAMINE	RIBOFLAVIN	NIACIN
Baked (1 potato)	202	145	4.0	0.2	32.8	1.1	31	0.15	0.07	2.7
Mashed (1 cup milk added)	210	137	4.4	1.5	27.3	0.8	21	0.17	0.11	2.1
French fries (frozen, reheated)	78	172	2.8	6.6	26.3	1.4	16	0.11	0.02	2.0
Dehydrated flakes (1 cup dry)	45	164	3.2	0.3	37.8	0.8	14	0.10	0.03	2.4
Dehydrated flakes (1 cup with milk, water, fat, salt)	210	195	4.0	6.7	30.5	0.6	11	0.08	0.08	1.9
Potato chips (10 chips)	20	114	1.1	8.0	10.0	0.4	3	0.04	0.01	1.0

231

Recommended Daily Allowances (RDAs) and Nutrient Values of Foods

Recommended Daily Dietary Allowances (RDAs) of Calories and Proteins

	AGE	POUNDS	HEIGHT	CALORIES NEEDED	GRAMS OF PROTEIN NEEDED
Males	11–14	97	63	2,800	44
	15–18	134	69	3,000	54
	19–22	147	69	3,000	54
	23–50	154	69	2,700	56
	51+	154	69	2,400	56
Females	11–14	97	62	2,400	44
	15–18	119	65	2,100	48
	19–22	128	65	2,100	46
	23–50	128	65	2,000	46
	51+	128	65	1,800	46
Pregnant				+300	+30
Nursing				+500	+20

Recommended Daily Allowances (RDAs) and Nutrient Values of Foods

Recommended Daily Dietary Allowances (RDAs) of Fat-Soluble Vitamins (in International Units)

	AGE	POUNDS	HEIGHT	VITAMIN A	VITAMIN D	VITAMIN E
Males	11–14	97	63	5,000	400	12
	15–18	134	69	5,000	400	15
	19–22	147	69	5,000	400	15
	23–50	154	69	5,000		15
	51+	154	69	5,000		15
Females	11–14	97	62	4,000	400	12
	15–18	119	65	4,000	400	12
	15–22	128	65	4,000	400	12
	23–50	128	65	4,000		12
	51+	128	65	4,000		12
Pregnant				5,000	400	15
Nursing				6,000	400	15

Appendix of Tables

Recommended Daily Dietary Allowances (RDAs) of Water-Soluble Vitamins (in Milligrams)

	AGE	POUNDS	HEIGHT	VITAMIN C	FOLIC ACID	NIACIN	RIBOFLAVIN	THIAMINE	VITAMIN B-6	VITAMIN B-12
Males	11–14	97	63	45	400	18	1.5	1.4	1.6	3.0
	15–18	134	69	45	400	20	1.8	1.5	2.0	3.0
	19–22	147	69	45	400	20	1.8	1.5	2.0	3.0
	23–50	154	69	45	400	18	1.6	1.4	2.0	3.0
	51+	154	69	45	400	16	1.5	1.2	2.0	3.0
Females	11–14	97	62	45	400	16	1.3	1.2	1.6	3.0
	15–18	119	65	45	400	14	1.4	1.1	2.0	3.0
	19–22	128	65	45	400	14	1.4	1.1	2.0	3.0
	23–50	128	65	45	400	13	1.2	1.0	2.0	3.0
	51+	128	65	45	400	12	1.1	1.0	2.0	3.0
Pregnant				60	800	+2	0.3	+0.3	2.5	4.0
Nursing				80	600	+4	+0.5	+0.3	2.5	4.0

Recommended Daily Allowances (RDAs) and Nutrient Values of Foods

Recommended Daily Dietary Allowances (RDAs) of Minerals (in Milligrams)

	AGE	POUNDS	HEIGHT	CALCIUM	PHOSPHORUS	IODINE	IRON	MAGNESIUM	ZINC
Males	11–14	97	63	1,200	1,200	130	18	350	15
	15–18	134	69	1,200	1,200	150	18	400	15
	19–22	147	69	800	800	140	10	350	15
	23–50	154	69	800	800	130	10	350	15
	51+	154	69	800	800	110	10	350	15
Females	11–14	97	62	1,200	1,200	115	18	300	15
	15–18	119	65	1,200	1,200	115	18	300	15
	19–22	128	65	800	800	100	18	300	15
	23–50	128	65	800	800	100	18	300	15
	51+	128	65	800	800	80	10	300	15
Pregnant				1,200	1,200	125	*18+	450	20
Nursing		1,200		150	18	450	25		

*A pregnant woman usually requires iron supplement tablets because of the difficulty in providing an adequate iron intake in an otherwise balanced diet.

235

Calcium Equivalents of Milk in Various Foods*

FOOD	CALCIUM (UNITS)
Evaporated milk, ½ cup	3.7
Cheese spread, 1⅞ oz.	17.1
Grated Parmesan cheese, 2½ tbsp.	10.7
Fresh skim milk, 1 cup	8.0
Buttermilk, 1 cup	4.0
Natural cheddar cheese, 1⅓ oz.	12.0
Process American cheese, 1½ oz.	10.7
Natural Swiss cheese, 1¼ oz.	12.8
Ice milk, 1½ cups	5.3
Ice cream, 1½ cups	5.3
Cheese food, 1⅞ oz.	4.3
Plain yogurt, 1 cup	0.8
Creamed cottage cheese, 1⅓ cups	3.0
Natural blue cheese, 3¼ oz.	1.2
Fruit-flavored yogurt, 1⅓ cups	0.6
Cream cheese, 17 oz.	0.5
Nonfat dry milk, ⅓ cup (dry)	48.0
Whole fluid milk, 1 cup	8.0

*1 cup of whole fluid milk equals 8 units.

Protein Equivalents of Various Food Sources*†

FOOD	AMOUNT (EQUAL TO 20G. PROTEIN)
Peanut Butter	4½ tbsp.
Enriched white bread	9 slices
Dry beans	1⅓ cups
Eggs (large)	3
Chicken	3 oz.
Canned bean soup	2½ cups
Whole milk	2⅓ cups
Ground beef	3 oz.
Beef liver	2⅔ oz.
Canned tuna (drained)	2½ oz.
Turkey	2¼ oz.
Processed American cheese	3 oz.
Cured ham	3⅓ oz.
Round beefsteak (lean)	2¼ oz.
Ocean perch fillet	3⅔ oz.
Pork chops (center cut)	2⅓ oz.
Bologna	6 oz.
Bacon	10 slices
Porterhouse steak (lean)	2⅓ oz.
Beef chuck roast (lean)	2½ oz.
Beef rump roast (lean)	2½ oz.

*The amount required to obtain 20 g. of protein.
†An adult man requires nearly 60 g. of protein daily; a pregnant woman or nursing mother requires about 70 g.

Nutrient Values of Various Cereals (per 3.5-oz. portion)

	CALORIES	PROTEIN (GRAMS)	FAT (G.)	CARBOHYDRATE (G.)	CALCIUM (MG.)	PHOSPHORUS (MG.)	IRON (MG.)	POTASSIUM (MG.)	THIAMINE (MG.)	RIBOFLAVIN (MG.)	NIACIN (MG.)
Barley, Scotch	348	9.6	1.1	77.2	34	290	2.7	296	.21	.07	3.7
Bran (40%) flakes (added thiamine)	303	10.2	1.8	80.6	71	495	4.4	—	.32	.13	5.3
Buckwheat, flour	333	11.7	2.5	72.0	33	347	2.8	—	.58	.15	2.9
Bulgur, dry	359	8.7	1.4	79.5	30	319	4.7	262	.30	.10	4.2
Corn, grits (dry, enriched)	362	8.7	0.8	78.1	4	73	2.9	80	.44	.26	3.5
Corn flakes (enriched)	386	7.9	0.4	85.3	17	45	1.4	120	.43	.08	2.1
Farina (dry, enriched)	371	11.4	0.9	77.0	25	107	2.9	83	.44	.26	3.5
Oats, rolled (dry)	390	14.2	7.4	68.2	53	405	4.5	352	.60	.14	1.0
Rice, brown	360	7.5	1.9	77.4	32	221	1.6	214	.34	.05	4.7
Rice, polished (instant, dry, enriched)	374	7.5	0.2	82.5	5	65	2.9	92	.44	.06	3.5
Rice, puffed (enriched)	390	5.9	0.3	87.7	29	132	1.6	180	.35	.05	5.4
Wheat, shredded	354	9.9	2.0	79.9	43	388	3.5	348	.22	.11	4.4
Wheat germ	363	26.6	10.9	46.7	72	1,118	9.4	827	2.01	.68	4.2
Whole-wheat flour	333	13.3	2.0	71.0	41	372	3.3	370	5.55	.12	4.3
Wild rice, raw	353	14.1	0.7	75.3	19	339	4.2	220	.45	.63	6.2

Appendix of Tables

Cholesterol Content of Various Foods*

FOOD	CHOLESTEROL (MILLIGRAMS)
1 cup skim milk	5
½ cup uncreamed cottage cheese	7
1 tbsp. lard	12
1 oz. light cream	20
½ cup creamed cottage cheese	24
¼ cup half-and-half	26
½ cup regular ice cream	27
1 oz. cheddar cheese	28
1 cup whole milk	34
1 tbsp. butter	35
3 oz. cooked salmon	40
3 oz. cooked oysters	40
3 oz. cooked clams	55
3 oz. cooked halibut or tuna	55
3 oz. cooked turkey or chicken (light meat)	67
3 oz. cooked beef, pork, or dark turkey meat	75
3 oz. cooked lamb or veal	85
3 oz. cooked shrimp	130
3 oz. beef heart	230
1 egg	250
3 oz. cooked beef, calf, or pork liver	370
3 oz. cooked kidney	680
3 oz. raw brains	1,700

*Given in milligrams per serving.

Fat Content and Major Fatty Acid Composition of Various Foods

FOOD	PERCENTAGE OF TOTAL FAT	PERCENTAGE OF: Saturated	Oleic	Unsaturated linoleic
Safflower oil	100	10	13	74
Sunflower oil	100	11	14	70
Corn oil	100	13	26	55
Cottonseed oil	100	23	17	54
Soybean oil	100	14	25	50
Sesame oil	100	14	38	42
Peanut oil	100	18	47	29
Olive oil	100	11	76	7
Coconut oil	100	80	5	1
Vegetable shortening	100	23	23	6–23
Safflower oil margarine	80	11	18	48

Fat Content and Major Fatty Acid Composition of Various Foods (continued)

FOOD	PERCENTAGE OF TOTAL FAT	Saturated	Oleic	Unsaturated linoleic
Corn oil margarine	80	14	26	38
Butter	81	46	27	2
Poultry fat	100	30	40	20
Beef, lamb, pork fat	100	45	44	2–6
Salmon, raw	9	2	2	4
Mackerel, raw	13	5	3	4
Pacific herring, raw	13	4	2	3
Tuna, raw	5	2	1	2
Egg yolk	31	10	13	2
Avocado	16	3	7	2
Peanut Butter	51	9	25	14
English walnuts	64	4	10	40
Black walnuts	60	4	21	28
Brazil nuts	67	13	32	17

Magnesium Content of Various Foods*

FOOD	MAGNESIUM (MILLIGRAMS)
Almonds	270
Barley, whole grain	124
Beans, white, dry	170
Beans, red, dry	163
Beans, lima, dry	180
Brazil nuts	225
Buckwheat, whole grain	229
Cashew nuts	267
Chocolate, sweet	107
Filberts	184
Molasses, blackstrap	258
Oats, rolled, dry	144
Peanuts, roasted, shelled	175
Peanut butter	173
Peas, dry	180
Rye, whole grain	115
Sesame seeds, raw	181
Soybeans, dry	265
Soybean curd (tofu)	111
Walnuts, black	190
Walnuts, English	131
Wheat, whole grain	160
Wheat germ	336
Wild rice	129
Yeast, Brewer's debittered	231

*Given in milligrams per 3.5-oz. serving. The U.S. RDA is 400 mg.

Appendix of Tables

Potassium Content of Various Foods*

FOOD	POTASSIUM (MILLIGRAMS)
Olives	55
Cheddar cheese	82
White bread	105
Canned crabmeat	110
Corn flakes	165
Chipped beef	200
Bacon	225
Frankfurter	230
Raw smoked ham	248
Salami	302
Canned salmon	330
Dried nonfat milk	1,335

*Given in milligrams per 3.5-oz. serving.

Sodium Content of Various Foods*

FOOD	SODIUM (MILLIGRAMS)
White bread	507
Dried nonfat milk	525
Canned salmon	540
Corn flakes	660
Cheddar cheese	700
Canned crabmeat	1,000
Frankfurter	1,100
Salami	1,260
Bacon	1,770
Olives	2,400
Raw smoked ham	2,530
Chipped beef	4,300
1 tsp. table salt	2,000

*Given in milligrams per 3.5-oz. serving.

Mineral and Vitamin Sources in Foods

Food Sources of Vitamin A*

FOOD	PERCENTAGE OF U.S. RDA	AMOUNT OF FOOD
Meat and Meat Alternates		
Liver, beef	910	3 oz.
Liver, calf	560	3 oz.
Liver, hog	250	3 oz.
Liver, chicken	60	1 oz.
Chicken or turkey potpie, home recipe	60	⅓ of 9-in. pie
Beef and vegetable stew	50	1 cup
Vegetables and Fruit		
Carrots, canned	470	1 cup
Sweet potatoes, mashed	400	1 cup
Carrots, cooked	330	1 cup
Spinach, canned	330	1 cup
Pumpkin, canned	310	1 cup
Sweet potatoes, pieces, canned	310	1 cup
Collards, cooked	300	1 cup
Peas and carrots, cooked	300	1 cup
Spinach, cooked	290	1 cup
Dandelion greens, cooked	250	1 cup
Carrots, raw, grated	240	1 cup
Sweet potatoes, boiled in skin	240	Medium potato
Turnip greens, canned, solids and liquid	220	1 cup
Cress, garden, cooked	210	1 cup
Chard, Swiss, cooked	190	1 cup
Mango, raw	190	1 fruit
Cantaloupe, raw	180	½ melon
Kale, cooked	180	1 cup
Mustard greens, cooked from frozen	180	1 cup
Sweet potatoes, baked in skin	180	Medium potato
Turnip greens, cooked	180	1 cup
Vegetables, mixed, cooked	180	1 cup
Squash, winter, baked	170	1 cup
Mustard greens, cooked	160	1 cup
Apricots, dried, cooked	150	1 cup
Beet greens, cooked	150	1 cup
Cabbage, spoon, cooked	110	1 cup

Appendix of Tables

Food Sources of Vitamin A* (continued)

FOOD	PERCENTAGE OF U.S. RDA	AMOUNT OF FOOD
Sweet potatoes, candied	110	3 oz. piece
Broccoli, chopped, cooked from frozen	100	1 cup
Apricots, canned	90	1 cup
Broccoli, cooked	90	Medium stalk
Spinach, raw, chopped	90	1 cup
Apricots, dried, uncooked	80	10 medium halves
Broccoli, cut, cooked	80	1 cup
Melon balls, frozen, in sirup	70	1 cup
Pepper, red	70	1 pod
Apricots, raw	60	3 fruits
Peaches, dried, cooked	60	1 cup
Plums, canned	60	1 cup
Carrots, strips, raw	60	6–8 strips
Papaya, raw, cubed	50	1 cup
Tomatoes, cooked	50	1 cup
Watermelon, raw	50	4 × 8-in. wedge
Cereal and Bakery Products		
Pie, pumpkin	80	4¾-in. sector
Pie, sweet potato	70	4¾-in. sector
Miscellaneous		
Soup:		
Vegetable, with beef broth	60	1 cup
Vegetable, vegetarian	60	1 cup
Vegetable beef	60	1 cup
Apricot nectar	50	1 cup

*Based on a U.S. RDA of 5,000 IU.

Food Sources of Thiamine (Vitamin B-1)*

FOOD	PERCENTAGE OF U.S. RDA	AMOUNT OF FOOD
Meat and Meat Alternates		
Sunflower seeds	190	1 cup
Pork, loin, chopped, lean	100	1 cup
Brazilnuts, shelled	90	1 cup

Food Sources of Thiamine (Vitamin B-1)* (continued)

FOOD	PERCENTAGE OF U.S. RDA	AMOUNT OF FOOD
Pork, fresh or cured, ham or shoulder, chopped, lean	60	1 cup
Pork, loin, sliced, lean	60	3 oz.
Pecans, halves	60	1 cup
Pork, loin chop, lean and fat	50	2.7 oz.
Pork, loin chop, lean	40	2 oz.
Cashew nuts, whole kernels, roasted	40	1 cup
Filberts, whole kernels, shelled	40	1 cup
Kidney, beef	30	3 oz.
Peanuts	30	1 cup
Spareribs	25	3 oz.
Spaghetti (enriched) with cheese, canned	25	1 cup
Cowpeas, dry, cooked	25	1 cup
Soybeans, dry, cooked	25	1 cup
Almonds, whole, shelled	25	1 cup
Chestnuts, shelled	25	1 cup
Pumpkin kernels	25	1 cup
Walnuts, English	25	1 cup
Liver, hog	20	3 oz.
Beef potpie, home prepared from enriched flour	20	⅓ of 9-in. pie
Chicken or turkey potpie, home prepared from enriched flour	20	⅓ of 9-in. pie
Chop suey, with beef and pork, home recipe	20	1 cup
Beans, navy (pea), dry, cooked	20	1 cup
Peas, split, dry, cooked	20	1 cup
Walnuts, black, chopped	20	1 cup
Bacon, Canadian	15	1 slice
Lamb, leg or shoulder, chopped, lean	15	1 cup
Heart, beef, sliced	15	3 oz.
Liver, calf or beef	15	3 oz.
Polish sausage	15	2.4 oz.
Pork sausage	15	1 oz.
Crab, deviled	15	1 cup
Lobster salad	15	A salad
Macaroni (enriched) and cheese, home recipe	15	1 cup
Spaghetti (enriched) with cheese, home recipe	15	1 cup
Spaghetti (enriched) with meatballs, home recipe	15	1 cup
Beans, canned, with pork and tomato sauce	15	1 cup
Beans, lima, Great Northern, or kidney, dry, cooked	15	1 cup

Appendix of Tables

Food Sources of Thiamine (Vitamin B-1)* (continued)

FOOD	PERCENTAGE OF U.S. RDA	AMOUNT OF FOOD
Vegetables and Fruit		
Cowpeas, cooked	35	1 cup
Peas, green, cooked	30	1 cup
Peas and carrots, cooked	20	1 cup
Beans, lima, fresh, cooked	20	1 cup
Asparagus, pieces, cooked	15	1 cup
Collards, cooked	15	1 cup
Cowpeas, canned, solids and liquid	15	1 cup
Okra, sliced, cooked	15	1 cup
Soybeans, sprouted seeds, raw or cooked	15	1 cup
Turnip greens, cooked	15	1 cup
Vegetables, mixed, cooked	15	1 cup
Potato salad, with cooked salad dressing	15	1 cup
Orange juice, fresh or from unsweetened frozen or canned concentrate	15	1 cup
Pineapple, canned, water or sirup pack	15	1 cup
Pineapple, frozen, sweetened	15	1 cup
Cereal and Bakery Products		
Hoagie roll, enriched	35	11½-in.-long roll
Cereal, ready to eat (check label)	25	1 oz.
Hard roll, enriched	15	1 roll (1.8 oz.)
Spoonbread	15	1 cup
Oatmeal, cooked	15	1 cup
Oat and wheat cereal, cooked	15	1 cup
Macaroni, enriched, cooked	15	1 cup
Noodles, enriched, cooked	15	1 cup
Spaghetti, enriched, cooked	15	1 cup
Rice, white, enriched, cooked	15	1 cup
Gingerbread, with enriched flour	15	1/9 of 9-in.-square cake
Pie, pecan	15	4¾-in. sector
Miscellaneous		
Orange juice, from dehydrated crystals	15	1 cup
Soup, split pea	15	1 cup
Bread pudding, with enriched bread	15	1 cup

*Based on a U.S. RDA of 1.5 mg.

Food Sources of Riboflavin (Vitamin B-2)*

FOOD	PERCENTAGE OF U.S. RDA	AMOUNT OF FOOD
Milk and Milk Products		
Cheese, cottage	35	1 cup
Milk, partially skimmed	30	1 cup
Malted beverage	30	1 cup
Custard, baked	30	1 cup
Milk, whole or skim	25	1 cup
Milk, nonfat dry, reconstituted	25	1 cup
Buttermilk	25	1 cup
Chocolate drink	25	1 cup
Cocoa	25	1 cup
Ice milk, soft serve	25	1 cup
Pudding, from mixes, with milk	25	1 cup
Pudding, vanilla, home recipe	25	1 cup
Rennin desserts	25	1 cup
Yogurt	25	1 cup
Ice cream, soft serve	20	1 cup
Pudding, chocolate, home recipe	20	1 cup
Tapioca cream	20	1 cup
Meat and Meat Alternates		
Kidney, beef	240	3 oz.
Liver, hog	220	3 oz.
Liver, beef or calf	210	3 oz.
Almonds, whole	80	1 cup
Fish loaf	60	4⅛ × 2½ × 1-in. slice
Heart, beef, sliced	60	3 oz.
Almonds, sliced	50	1 cup
Liver, chicken	40	1 oz.
Beef, dried, chipped, creamed	30	1 cup
Welsh rarebit	30	1 cup
Lamb, leg or shoulder, chopped, lean	25	1 cup
Pork, fresh, ham or loin, chopped, lean	25	1 cup
Veal, stewed or roasted, chopped	25	1 cup
Braunschweiger	25	1 oz.
Chicken a la king, home recipe	25	1 cup
Macaroni (enriched) and cheese, home recipe	25	1 cup
Beef, chuck or rump, chopped, lean	20	1 cup
Lamb, leg or shoulder, chopped, lean and fat	20	1 cup
Pork, cured, ham or shoulder, chopped, lean	20	1 cup
Pork, fresh, shoulder, chopped	20	1 cup

Appendix of Tables

Food Sources of Riboflavin (Vitamin B-2)* (continued)

FOOD	PERCENTAGE OF U.S. RDA	AMOUNT OF FOOD
Pork, fresh, ham or shoulder, ground, lean	20	1 cup
Veal, loin, chopped	20	1 cup
Veal, rib, ground	20	1 cup
Turkey, dark meat, chopped	20	1 cup
Chicken or turkey potpie, home prepared from enriched flour	30	⅓ of 9-in. pie
Chop suey with beef and pork, home recipe	20	1 cup
Pepper, stuffed	20	1 pepper (6.5 oz.)
Spaghetti (enriched) with meatballs, home recipe	20	1 cup
Vegetables and Fruit		
Broccoli, cooked	20	Medium stalk
Broccoli, cut, cooked	20	1 cup
Corn pudding	20	1 cup
Collards, cooked	20	1 cup
Turnip greens, cooked	20	1 cup
Avocado, Florida, raw	20	½ fruit
Avocado, Florida or California, raw, cubed	20	1 cup
Cereal and Bakery Products		
Cereals, ready to eat (check label)	25	1 oz.
Spoonbread	25	1 cup
Hoagie roll, enriched	20	11½-in.-long roll
Miscellaneous		
Bread pudding, with enriched bread	35	1 cup
Oyster stew, home recipe	25	1 cup
Rice pudding	20	1 cup
Soup, cream of mushroom, with milk	20	1 cup

*Based on a U.S. RDA of 1.7 mg.

Mineral and Vitamin Sources in Foods

Food Sources of Vitamin C*

FOOD	PERCENTAGE OF U.S. RDA	AMOUNT OF FOOD
Meat and Meat Alternates		
Peppers, stuffed	120	1 pepper
Lobster salad	80	A salad
Chop suey, with beef and pork, home recipe	60	1 cup
Liver, calf	50	3 oz.
Vegetables and Fruit		
Broccoli, cooked	270	Medium stalk
Pepper, red, raw	250	1 pod
Collards, cooked	240	1 cup
Broccoli, cut, cooked	230	1 cup
Brussels sprouts, cooked	230	1 cup
Strawberries, frozen, sweetened	230	1 cup
Pepper, green, cooked	220	1 cup
Orange juice, fresh	210	1 cup
Orange juice, from frozen or canned concentrate	200	1 cup
Broccoli, chopped, cooked from frozen	180	1 cup
Kale, cooked	170	1 cup
Turnip greens, cooked	170	1 cup
Orange juice, canned	170	1 cup
Peaches, frozen	170	1 cup
Pepper, green, raw	160	1 pod
Grapefruit juice, fresh or from frozen unsweetened concentrate	160	1 cup
Cantaloup, raw	150	½ melon
Orange sections, raw	150	1 cup
Strawberries, raw	150	1 cup
Grapefruit sections, raw, white or pink	140	1 cup
Grapefruit juice, canned, unsweetened	140	1 cup
Grapefruit juice, from frozen sweetened concentrate	140	1 cup
Grapefruit sections, canned, sirup pack	130	1 cup
Grapefruit juice, canned, sweetened	130	1 cup
Papaya, raw, cubed	130	1 cup
Grapefruit sections, canned, water pack	120	1 cup
Mango, raw	120	1 fruit (⅔ lb.)
Cauliflower, cooked	120	1 cup
Cauliflower, raw	110	1 cup
Mustard greens, cooked	110	1 cup
Orange, raw	110	2⅝-in.-diameter orange

247

Appendix of Tables

Food Sources of Vitamin C* (continued)

FOOD	PERCENTAGE OF U.S. RDA	AMOUNT OF FOOD
Tangerine juice, from frozen concentrate	110	1 cup
Tomatoes, cooked	100	1 cup
Raspberries, red, frozen	90	1 cup
Tangerine juice, canned	90	1 cup
Cabbage, cooked	80	1 cup
Cress, garden, cooked	80	1 cup
Spinach, cooked	80	1 cup
Strawberries, canned	80	1 cup
Cabbage, raw, finely shredded	70	1 cup
Cabbage, red, raw, shredded	70	1 cup
Rutabagas, cooked	70	1 cup
Tomatoes, raw	70	3-in.-diameter tomato
Turnip greens, canned, solids and liquid	70	1 cup
Tomato juice, canned or bottled	70	1 cup
Sauerkraut juice	70	1 cup
Grapefruit, white or pink, raw	70	½ medium fruit
Lemons, raw	70	1 lemon
Asparagus, pieces, cooked or canned	60	1 cup
Cabbage, common or savoy, raw, coarsely shredded	60	1 cup
Okra, sliced, cooked	60	1 cup
Peas, green, cooked	60	1 cup
Sauerkraut, canned	60	1 cup
Sweet potatoes, canned, mashed	60	1 cup
Turnips, cooked	60	1 cup
Coleslaw	60	1 cup
Honeydew melon, raw	60	2 × 7-in. wedge
Loganberries, raw	60	1 cup
Melon balls, frozen, sirup pack	60	1 cup
Beans, lima, Fordhook, cooked from frozen	50	1 cup
Beans, lima, immature seeds, cooked	50	1 cup
Mustard greens, cooked from frozen	50	1 cup
Potato, baked in skin	50	Medium potato
Spinach, canned	50	1 cup
Blackberries, raw	50	1 cup
Raspberries, red, raw	50	1 cup
Watermelon, raw	50	4 × 8-in. wedge
Pineapple juice, from frozen concentrate	50	1 cup

Mineral and Vitamin Sources in Foods

Food Sources of Vitamin C* (continued)

FOOD	PERCENTAGE OF U.S. RDA	AMOUNT OF FOOD
Cereal and Bakery Products		
Spanish rice	60	1 cup
Pie, strawberry	50	4¾-in.-sector
Miscellaneous		
Orange juice, from dehydrated crystals	180	1 cup
Grapefruit juice, from dehydrated crystals	150	1 cup
Cranberry juice cocktail	70	1 cup
Grape juice drink, canned	70	1 cup
Orange-apricot juice drink	70	1 cup
Pineapple-orange juice drink	70	1 cup
Pineapple-grapefruit juice drink	70	1 cup

*Based on a U.S. RDA of 60 mg.

Food Sources of Calcium*

FOOD	PERCENTAGE OF U.S. RDA	AMOUNT OF FOOD
Milk and Milk Products		
Cheese, Parmesan, grated	40	1 oz.
Milk, partially skimmed	35	1 cup
Pudding, uncooked, from mix	35	1 cup
Milk, whole or skim	30	1 cup
Milk, nonfat dry, reconstituted	30	1 cup
Buttermilk	30	1 cup
Chocolate drink, made from whole milk	30	1 cup
Cocoa	30	1 cup
Malted beverage	30	1 cup
Custard, baked	30	1 cup
Pudding, vanilla, home recipe	30	1 cup
Rennin desserts	30	1 cup
Yogurt, made from partially skimmed milk	30	1 cup
Chocolate drink, made from skim milk	25	1 cup
Cheese, cottage, creamed	25	1 cup
Cheese, Swiss	25	1 oz.
Yogurt, made from whole milk	25	1 cup
Ice cream or ice milk, soft serve	25	1 cup
Pudding, cooked, from mix, with milk	25	1 cup
Pudding, chocolate, home recipe	25	1 cup
Cheese, American, processed	20	1 oz.

Appendix of Tables

Food Sources of Calcium* (continued)

FOOD	PERCENTAGE OF U.S. RDA	AMOUNT OF FOOD
Cheese, Cheddar, natural	20	1 oz.
Cheese, cottage, uncreamed	20	1 cup
Ice cream or ice milk, hardened	20	1 cup
Meat and Meat Alternates		
Welsh rarebit	60	1 cup
Sardines, canned, drained	35	3 oz.
Macaroni (enriched) and cheese, home recipe	35	1 cup
Potatoes au gratin	30	1 cup
Beef, dried, chipped, creamed	25	1 cup
Cheese souffle	20	1 cup
Lobster Newburg	20	1 cup
Macaroni (enriched) and cheese, canned	20	1 cup
Vegetables and Fruit		
Collards, cooked	35	1 cup
Cabbage, spoon, cooked	25	1 cup
Spinach, canned	25	1 cup
Turnip greens	25	1 cup
Kale, cooked	20	1 cup
Mustard greens, cooked	20	1 cup
Rhubarb, cooked	20	1 cup
Cereal and Bakery Products		
Spoonbread	25	1 cup
Farina, enriched, instant	20	1 cup
Miscellaneous		
Bread pudding	30	1 cup
Oyster stew, home recipe	30	1 cup
Rice pudding	25	1 oup
Soup, with milk:		
Green pea	20	1 cup
Cream of celery	20	1 cup
Cream of mushroom	20	1 cup
Cream of asparagus	20	1 cup

*Based on a U.S. RDA of 1 g.

Mineral and Vitamin Sources in Foods

Food Sources of Iron*

FOOD	PERCENTAGE OF U.S. RDA	AMOUNT OF FOOD
Meat and Meat Alternates		
Liver, hog	140	3 oz.
Pumpkin kernels	90	1 cup
Liver, calf	70	3 oz.
Kidney, beef	60	3 oz.
Sunflower seeds	60	1 cup
Liver, beef	40	3 oz.
Walnuts, black, chopped	40	1 cup
Clams, canned, drained, chopped	35	1 cup
Beans, lima, dry, cooked	35	1 cup
Beans, with pork and sweet sauce, canned	35	1 cup
Almonds, whole, shelled	35	1 cup
Beef, chuck or rump, chopped, lean	30	1 cup
Pork, cured, shoulder, chopped, lean	30	1 cup
Pork, fresh, ham or loin, chopped, lean	30	1 cup
Heart, beef, sliced	30	3 oz.
Clams, raw	30	4 or 5 clams
Beef potpie, home prepared from enriched flour	30	⅓ of 9-in. pie
Beans, navy (pea), dry, cooked	30	1 cup
Beans, white, dry, canned, solids and liquid	30	1 cup
Cashew nuts, whole kernels, roasted	30	1 cup
Beef, chuck or rump, ground, lean	25	1 cup
Pork, cured, ham, chopped, lean	25	1 cup
Pork, fresh, shoulder, chopped	25	1 cup
Pork, fresh, ham, ground, lean	25	1 cup
Veal, chopped	25	1 cup
Chicken or turkey potpie, home prepared from enriched flour	25	⅓ of 9-in. pie
Chile con carne with beans, canned	25	1 cup
Chop suey, with beef and pork, home recipe	25	1 cup
Corned beef hash, canned	25	1 cup
Beans, Great Northern or red kidney, dry, cooked	25	1 cup
Beans, red kidney, dry, canned, solids and liquid	25	1 cup
Lentils, dry, cooked	25	1 cup
Soybeans, dry, cooked	25	1 cup
Beans, with frankfurters, canned	25	1 cup
Beans, with pork and tomato sauce, canned	25	1 cup
Beef, chuck, sliced, lean	20	3 oz.
Beef, flank steak	20	3 oz.

Appendix of Tables

Food Sources of Iron* (continued)

FOOD	PERCENTAGE OF U.S. RDA	AMOUNT OF FOOD
Beef, plate, lean	20	3 oz.
Beef, steak, sirloin, lean	20	3 oz.
Pork, cured, ham or shoulder, ground, lean	20	1 cup
Pork, fresh, shoulder, ground, lean	20	1 cup
Pork, fresh, ham, sliced, lean	20	3 oz.
Pork, loin, sliced, lean	20	3 oz.
Turkey, dark meat, chopped	20	1 cup
Peppers, stuffed	20	1 pepper (6.5 oz.)
Spaghetti (enriched) in tomato sauce, with meatballs; canned or home prepared	20	1 cup
Cowpeas, dry, cooked	20	1 cup
Peas, split, dry, cooked	20	1 cup
Beef, chuck, lean and fat, sliced	15	3 oz.
Beef, corned	15	3 oz.
Beef, plate, lean and fat	15	3 oz.
Beef, rump, sliced	15	3 oz.
Beef, rib, sliced, lean	15	3 oz.
Beef, steak (round)	15	3 oz.
Beef, steak (club, porterhouse, or T-bone), lean	15	3 oz.
Beef, steak (sirloin), lean and fat	15	3 oz.
Ground beef	15	3 oz.
Lamb, shoulder, chopped, lean	15	1 cup
Lamb, leg, chopped	15	1 cup
Pork, cured, shoulder, sliced	15	3 oz.
Pork, cured, ham, sliced, lean	15	3 oz.
Pork, fresh, loin or ham, sliced, lean and fat	15	3 oz.
Pork, loin chop, lean and fat	15	2.7 oz.
Pork, fresh, shoulder, sliced	15	3 oz.
Veal, sliced	15	3 oz.
Veal, cutlet or loin	15	3 oz.
Beef and vegetable stew, home recipe	15	1 cup
Chicken, dark meat, chopped	15	1 cup
Chicken, canned	15	1 cup
Spaghetti (enriched) with tomato sauce and cheese, canned	15	1 cup
Turkey, canned	15	1 cup
Chow mein, chicken, home recipe	15	1 cup
Chicken a la king, home recipe	15	1 cup
Crab, deviled	15	1 cup
Sardines, canned	15	3 oz.
Shrimp, canned	15	3 oz.
Lobster salad	15	A salad
Tuna salad	15	1 cup

Food Sources of Iron* (continued)

FOOD	PERCENTAGE OF U.S. RDA	AMOUNT OF FOOD
Vegetables and Fruit		
Peaches, dried, uncooked	60	1 cup
Prune juice, canned	60	1 cup
Dates, pitted, chopped	30	1 cup
Raisins, seedless	30	1 cup
Spinach, canned	30	1 cup
Asparagus, pieces, canned	25	1 cup
Beans, lima, canned	25	1 cup
Beans, lima, fresh or frozen, baby, cooked	25	1 cup
Apricots, dried, cooked	25	1 cup
Peaches, dried, cooked	25	1 cup
Cowpeas, cooked	20	1 cup
Cowpeas, canned, solids and liquid	20	1 cup
Peas, green, canned	20	1 cup
Spinach, cooked	20	1 cup
Turnip greens, canned, solids and liquid	20	1 cup
Prunes, dried, cooked	20	1 cup
Beans, lima, Fordhook, cooked	15	1 cup
Beet greens, cooked	15	1 cup
Chard, Swiss, cooked	15	1 cup
Mustard greens, fresh or frozen, cooked	15	1 cup
Peas, green, cooked	15	1 cup
Sauerkraut juice	15	1 cup
Vegetables, mixed, cooked	15	1 cup
Boysenberries, canned	15	1 cup
Plums, canned, water or sirup pack	15	1 cup
Prunes, dried, uncooked	15	10 prunes
Cereal and Bakery Products		
Farina, instant, enriched, cooked	90	1 cup
Farina, regular and quick cooking, enriched, cooked	70	1 cup
Hoagie roll, enriched	40	11½-in.-long roll
Cereals, ready to eat (check label)	20	1 oz.
Cottage pudding with enriched flour and chocolate sauce	20	1/6 of 8-in.-square cake
Gingerbread, with enriched flour	20	1/9 of 8-in.-square cake
Pie, pecan	20	4¾-in. sector
Coffeecake, with enriched flour	15	2.5-oz. piece

Appendix of Tables

Food Sources of Iron* (continued)

FOOD	PERCENTAGE OF U.S. RDA	AMOUNT OF FOOD
Cottage pudding, with enriched flour and strawberry sauce	15	1/6 of 8-in.-square cake
Hard roll, enriched	15	1 roll (1.8 oz.)
Spoonbread	15	1 cup
Miscellaneous		
Bread pudding, with raisins and enriched bread	20	1 cup
Oyster stew, home recipe	20	1 cup
Molasses, blackstrap	20	1 tbsp.
Apple brown betty, with enriched bread	15	1 cup
Sirup, sorghum	15	1 tbsp.

*Based on a U.S. RDA of 18 mg.

Food Sources of Niacin (Nicotinic Acid)*

FOOD	PERCENTAGE OF U.S. RDA	AMOUNT OF FOOD
Meat and Meat Alternates		
Peanuts	120	1 cup
Liver, hog	100	3 oz.
Chicken, light meat, chopped	80	1 cup
Turkey, light meat, chopped	80	1 cup
Liver, calf or beef	70	3 oz.
Chicken, breast	60	½ breast (3.3 oz.)
Chicken, stewed, dark meat, chopped	60	1 cup
Veal rib, chopped	60	1 cup
Tuna, canned in water	60	3 oz.
Chicken, roasted, light meat, sliced	50	3 oz.
Turkey, canned	50	1 cup
Rabbit, domesticated	50	3 oz.
Tuna, canned in oil, drained	50	3 oz.
Tuna salad	50	1 cup
Lamb, leg, chopped, lean	45	1 cup
Kidney, beef	45	3 oz.
Pork, loin, chopped, lean	45	1 cup
Veal, stewed, chopped	45	1 cup
Veal, rib, ground	45	1 cup
Chicken, canned	45	1 cup
Chicken, stewed, light meat, sliced	45	3 oz.

Food Sources of Niacin (Nicotinic Acid)* (continued)

FOOD	PERCENTAGE OF U.S. RDA	AMOUNT OF FOOD
Turkey, light meat, sliced	45	3 oz.
Swordfish, broiled	45	3 oz.
Chicken, broiled	40	3 oz.
Goose	40	3 oz.
Lamb, shoulder, chopped, lean	40	1 cup
Pork, fresh, ham, chopped, lean	40	1 cup
Veal, loin, chopped	40	1 cup
Turkey potpie, home prepared from enriched flour	40	⅓ of 9-in. pie
Salmon steak, broiled or baked	40	3 oz.
Sunflower seeds	40	1 cup
Beef, rump, chopped, lean	35	1 cup
Pork, fresh or cured, shoulder, chopped, lean	35	1 cup
Veal, rib, sliced	35	3 oz.
Heart, beef, sliced	35	3 oz.
Chicken, stewed, dark meat, sliced	35	3 oz.
Chicken, roasted, dark meat, chopped	35	1 cup
Halibut, broiled	35	3 oz.
Mackerel, broiled	35	3 oz.
Rockfish, oven steamed	35	3 oz.
Shad, baked	35	3 oz.
Beef, chuck, chopped	30	1 cup
Beef, rump, ground, lean	30	1 cup
Pork, cured, ham, chopped, lean	30	1 cup
Pork, cured, shoulder, ground, lean	30	1 cup
Pork, loin, sliced, lean	30	3 oz.
Chicken fricassee, home recipe	30	1 cup
Turkey, dark meat, chopped	30	1 cup
Salmon, pink, canned	30	3 oz.
Beef potpie, home prepared from flour	30	⅓ of 9-in. pie
Beef, chuck, ground, lean	25	1 cup
Beef, steak (club, porterhouse, T-bone, or sirloin), lean	25	3 oz.
Beef, steak (round)	25	3 oz.
Ground beef	25	3 oz.
Lamb, leg, sliced	25	3 oz.
Lamb, loin chop, lean and fat	25	3.5 oz.
Lamb, shoulder, sliced, lean	25	3 oz.
Pork, cured, ham, ground, lean	25	3 oz.
Pork, fresh, ham, sliced, lean	25	3 oz.
Pork, loin chop, lean and fat	25	2.7 oz.
Pork, loin, sliced, lean and fat	25	3 oz.
Veal, stewed, sliced	25	3 oz.

Appendix of Tables

Food Sources of Niacin (Nicotinic Acid)* (continued)

FOOD	PERCENTAGE OF U.S. RDA	AMOUNT OF FOOD
Veal, loin or cutlet	25	3 oz.
Chicken, roasted, dark meat, sliced	25	3 oz.
Chicken a la king, home recipe	25	1 cup
Chicken potpie, home prepared from enriched flour	25	⅓ of 9-in. pie
Salmon, red, canned	25	3 oz.
Salmon rice loaf	25	6-oz. piece
Sardines, canned, drained	25	3 oz.
Beef and vegetable stew, home recipe	25	1 cup
Chop suey, with beef and pork, home recipe	25	1 cup
Corned beef hash, canned	25	1 cup
Peppers, stuffed	25	1 pepper
Spaghetti (enriched) with cheese, canned	25	1 cup
Beef, chuck, sliced	20	3 oz.
Beef, rump, sliced	20	3 oz.
Beef, rib, sliced, lean and fat	20	3 oz.
Beef, flank steak	20	3 oz.
Beef, plate, lean	20	3 oz.
Beef, steak (club, porterhouse, T-bone, or sirloin), lean and fat	20	3 oz.
Lamb, rib chop, lean and fat	20	3.2 oz.
Lamb, loin chop, lean	20	2.3 oz.
Lamb, shoulder, sliced, lean and fat	20	3 oz.
Pork, cured, ham, sliced, lean	20	3 oz.
Pork, fresh, ham, sliced, lean and fat	20	3 oz.
Pork, fresh or cured, shoulder, sliced	20	3 oz.
Pork, loin chop, lean	20	2 oz.
Chicken, thigh	20	2.3-oz. piece
Turkey, dark meat, sliced	20	3 oz.
Chicken and noodles, home recipe	20	1 cup
Chow mein, home recipe	20	1 cup
Spaghetti (enriched) with meatballs, home recipe	20	1 cup
Lobster salad	20	A salad
Lobster Newburg	20	1 cup
Crab, deviled	20	1 cup
Vegetables and Fruits		
Dates, pitted, chopped	20	1 cup
Peaches, dried, cooked, unsweetened	20	1 cup
Peas, green, cooked	20	1 cup

Mineral and Vitamin Sources in Foods

Food Sources of Niacin (Nicotinic Acid)* (continued)

FOOD	PERCENTAGE OF U.S. RDA	AMOUNT OF FOOD
Cereal and Bakery Products		
Hoagie roll, enriched	25	11½-in. long roll
Cereals, ready to eat (check label)	20	1 oz.

*Based on a U.S. RDA of 20 mg.

A000013843137